CONTENTS

INTRODUCTION

D o you desire to be healthy? Do you desire to have beneficial and lasting relationships? Do you long to be free from the baggage of your past and the resentment, guilt, and shame that it brings? Do you wish to break free from the negative thoughts that have plagued you for so long? Do you desire to have power in your life to unshackle yourself from those habits that have held you in chains?

If this is your desire, this book is for you. In this book, we are going to explore together The Law of Life. The Law of Life, applied in your life and functioning in your heart, can bring you a power and freedom that you always searched for but never found. It is liberating in concept but challenging in application. It calls for everything you have but offers what you don't. It is comprehensive but easily understood. It is simple but profound.

This book was not written in the typical style of a book, because it is, in reality, a transcript of a lecture series. As I developed this lecture series and it began to grow, audiences asked me for notes so that they could study further into the topics that I was presenting. At first, the notes were only a few pages long. But within a year, they filled 25 pages of letter-sized paper, wide margin, single-spaced.

It was at that point that I decided it would be better to turn the notes into a small booklet to accompany the lectures. Over the last few years, the booklet has continued to grow, but has remained in the transcript format. The illustrations are taken directly from my PowerPoint slides so that you can have a visual reference as you read about a topic.

If you would like to view the actual lecture series, there are several iterations of The Law of Life series on Uchee Pines Institute's

YouTube channel. These can be accessed at the following link: https://www.youtube.com/UcheePinesInstitute

I recommend reading the book through at least 6-10 times. Each time you read it, you will catch new information that you missed previously, and principles and concepts will come together in your mind in new ways.

May you find the freedom and power that you are looking for as you diligently read, study, and apply the principles of The Law of Life in your own life.

CHAPTER ONE

Understanding the Cause of Disease

Treating the Cause

I n this series, we want to talk about treating the cause of disease, not just its symptoms. But in order to treat the cause, we must know what the cause is. What is the cause of disease? What is the cause of cancer? What is the cause of diabetes? What is the cause of coronary artery disease? What is the cause of auto-immune diseases?

Don't feel bad if you don't have an answer to these questions. If you were to go to your doctor and ask them, "What is the cause of my disease?" they will give you a list of risk factors that are known to be associated with your disease condition. But if you keep asking them what the foundational cause of your disease is—that thing that would allow you to recover if it were removed—they would not be able to tell you. They don't know.

But if you don't know the cause, how can you successfully treat and remove it? This is why I am interested in causes.

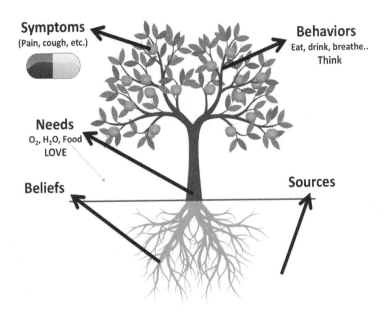

Of Trees and Men

There are many similarities between people and plants. And when it comes to health, we can better understand ourselves and how we gain and maintain health by comparing ourselves with trees.

Imagine that you have a fruit tree and it is fruit season. What are some of the first things that you notice about the tree? The fruit and the leaves and the shape of the tree? In this analogy, the fruit and the leaves represent our symptoms. These are the obvious things we notice and complain about, like pain, coughing, itching, etc.

If you have a tree that has some bad fruit and bad leaves, does it solve the problem to pluck off the bad fruit and leaves? No. Plucking off the bad fruit and bad leaves only removes the evidence of the problem, but it doesn't solve the problem. If you have pain in your back and you go to your doctor and your doctor gives you a pill to decrease the pain, you feel better. But the pain is still there. So, you go to doctor number 2 and 3, and get more pills. Eventually, you don't have any more pain. Your problem is solved, right? No. You have only removed the manifestation of the problem, but not the problem itself.

Let us assume that you go to a fourth doctor, and this doctor does an examination and finds that you have a knife stuck in your back! Did the pain pills remove the cause? No. They only masked its manifestation. This is similar to having your house on fire and solving the problem by turning off the fire alarm. Treating the symptoms will not fix the problem, it will only limit its manifestation.

I don't want you to think that symptom care is never appropriate. If I break a bone or cut off a finger, please give me something to deal with the pain! But don't just treat the pain. Fix the problem as well.

Why does it not fix the problem to pluck off the bad fruit and bad leaves? It is because the fruit and leaves do not support themselves. They are supported by the branches, and the branches represent our behaviors or actions. These actions or behaviors are simple things like breathing, eating, drinking, exposing, sleeping, etc.

If the tree has healthy branches, they will support healthy leaves and fruit. But if the tree has unhealthy branches, they will promote diseased fruit and leaves. Similarly, if your behaviors are good, they will support good symptoms, but if your behaviors are bad, they will promote bad symptoms.

If the tree has unhealthy branches, will it help the problem to prune the branches? Yes, it will. It can decrease the disease burden. But it doesn't solve the problem, because the problem is ultimately not in the branches, because the branches don't support themselves. They are supported by the trunk, and the trunk represents our needs.

You need what you need because you are what you are. We, as human beings, need oxygen, water, food, sunlight, warmth, rest, etc. You and I can't change what we need, because those needs are determined by what we are. Trees have different needs than reptiles, which have different needs than birds, which have different needs than humans. And what we need and how much of it we need is determined by what we are.

What you need is internal—it is determined by what you are. But the source of what you need is external—it lies outside of you and must be brought in from the outside and incorporated into yourself. You need oxygen, but the oxygen you need is outside of yourself and must be brought in in order for you to live. You need water, but the water you need is outside of yourself and must be brought in in order for you to live. You need food, but the food you need is outside of yourself and must be brought in in order for you to live.

Everything you need, which is determined by what you are, must be actively brought in to you from the outside. And your behaviors (breathing, drinking, eating, etc.) are the actions that bring in to you what you need from outside.

If your behaviors match your needs, you will promote good symptoms, just as branches that correctly transport the sap from the trunk promote healthy leaves and fruit. But if your behaviors do not match your needs, then you will promote bad symptoms, just as branches that do not correctly transport the sap from the trunk will promote diseased leaves and fruit.

For example, you need a certain amount of water daily to remain properly hydrated. If you drink a sufficient amount of water to remain properly hydrated, that will promote good symptoms. But if don't drink a sufficient amount of water, if your actions do not match your needs, you will end up with symptoms of headache, fatigue, dry lips, constipation, etc.

If you have diseased fruit and leaves on your tree, I don't know of anything that you can do to the trunk of the tree to fix the problem. You can cut if off, but otherwise, there is little that you can do with the trunk. To really get to the problem, you need to go underground. Why? Because the trunk doesn't support itself. It is supported by the roots, and the roots represent our beliefs.

So far, we have been dealing with aspects that are pretty obvious (above the ground). Symptoms are obvious. Behaviors are obvious. Needs are fairly obvious. But beliefs? In order to know what someone believes you need to dig a bit. But, although you need to dig a bit, be sure that the roots affect the health of the branches. You do what you do because you believe what you believe.

If your beliefs about what you need match with your actual needs, then your behaviors will match your needs as well, and this will promote healthy fruit and leaves. But if your beliefs about what you need do not match with your actual needs, this will promote diseased fruit and leaves.

For example, let us imagine that you believe you *need* Coca Cola. If you believe you need Coca Cola, you will drink Coca Cola. But do you actually need Coca Cola? No! If you supply something that you don't need, or if you don't supply what you do need, this will promote diseased fruit and leaves—bad symptoms. It is only as you believe correctly about what you need so that you behave correctly in supplying what you need that you can expect healthy fruit and leaves, or good symptoms.

But as yet, there is something missing. You see, when the tree has bad fruit and bad leaves, it is rarely the tree that is the problem. There is not a lot of surgery that an arborist does to the roots of the tree if the tree is struggling. Sure, if it is root-bound, the roots can be separated and spread out. But there isn't a lot to do with the roots. What does the arborist fix if the tree has a problem? They fix the soil! You see, the problem is not so much in the tree as it is in the soil. And the soil represents our sources.

If you believe that you need water and you drink water, but the water you drink is polluted, that will still promote diseased fruit and leaves. But, if you believe that you need water and you drink a sufficient amount of pure water, that will promote healthy leaves and fruit—good symptoms.

So, healthy fruit and leaves are the product of good sources, beliefs that match with one's needs, and behaviors that correctly supply those needs. When all of these are working together, one can expect health and good symptoms.

In a human, however, there is at least one more aspect that we must consider. In a tree, the roots cannot choose what source to take from. It simply takes from that which is around it. However, a functional, adult human, can choose its source. And the choices of what sources we take from are also rooted upon our beliefs. So, not only do the beliefs determine the behaviors, but the beliefs determine the sources we take from. This will become clearer as we continue through this series. But for now, just remember: if you see bad fruit on your tree, don't pluck off the fruit. Dig in the ground to find out what is going on with the roots and the soil. That is where you will find the cause of your disease.

I have a question for you. Do you need love? Is there anyone here that does not need love? I have asked this question to thousands of people around the world, and I have not found a single person that does not need love. We all need love, just like we all need oxygen, water, food, etc.

Our need of love is determined by what we are—human beings. And the source of the love that we need is outside of ourselves, just as the source of the oxygen, water, and food that we need is outside of ourselves. And like the oxygen, water, and food, there must be an action that brings the love in to us so that we can live. And what is that action? It is thinking. Thinking is the action that brings in the love that we need in order to survive.

Is it possible that love is just like the other needs; that there can be a polluted or a good source; that there can be correct or false beliefs about love; and that there can be appropriate actions (thinking) that fulfill that need, or inappropriate actions that do not fulfill that need? And if the source, beliefs, or actions (thoughts) are not right, there can be diseased fruit and leaves, but if the source, beliefs, or actions are right, there can be healthy fruit and leaves? Yes, this is the case. But we will dive into this topic further later in this book.

Pain & Disease

How many of you like pain? And how many like disease? I have a question for you. Is the function of pain and disease a good function or a bad function? Let us take leprosy for an example.

In leprosy, individuals are infected with a type of bacteria that begins affecting areas of the body which are cool, like the fingers, toes, and nose. The infection damages the nerves and eventually a person is not able to feel. Then, when something harmful happens to their hands or feet, they can't feel it, so they eventually start losing their fingers and toes because of injuries, burns, cuts, and other problems which they can't feel. If you and I put our hand on the burner, we will pull it off right away because we feel pain. They don't pull their hand off the burner until they smell the flesh burning, because they can't feel.

So, is the function of pain good? Is it good to have the capacity to feel pain? Yes! Similarly, is the function of disease good? Is it good to have the capacity to have disease? Yes. Both pain and disease let us know that something is wrong. If we didn't have that capacity, we would injure ourselves beyond repair in a very short period of time.

But as we look a little closer at disease, we need to ask ourselves a question. Does disease just come out of thin air, or is there a cause to disease? If disease has a cause, what is it? In order to help us come to an understanding of the cause of disease, we must begin reasoning from cause to effect, or from an effect back to the cause.

The Law of Cause and Effect (Hypertension Example)

Let us take hypertension, or high blood pressure, for our example. What is the cause of high blood pressure? We know that when the blood vessels clamp down on the blood that is within them, the pressure of the blood (blood pressure) increases. So, vasoconstriction is the cause of high blood pressure. We've solved the problem, right? We've found the cause of high blood pressure, right?

A colleague of mine has this to say: "Causes have causes." Just because we find one cause to a problem doesn't mean we have found THE cause. Each cause we find is caused by something else, until we get to the root cause.

So, in the case of vasoconstriction, we find that it is the result of increased activity of the sympathetic nervous system, which is your fight or flight response system. It causes the heart rate to increase, the blood vessels to clamp down, and a large release of adrenaline, which all increases your blood pressure. But what is the cause of increased sympathetic nervous system stimulation?

One of the causes is increased leptin. Leptin is a hormone that is released from the fat cells in the body (predominantly the fat that is around the organs in the abdomen), and this hormone travels in the blood to a part of the brain called the hypothalamus, which has receptors in it for leptin. When there is more leptin coming to the hypothalamus, it triggers the sympathetic nervous system to increase its output. But what is the cause of increased leptin?

It is increased fat in the body, especially central fat around the organs. The fat cells primarily grow in size as one gains weight, and as the cells get bigger and bigger, it is harder for nutrients and gasses to dissolve to the center part of the cell. In defense, the cells release leptin, and the leptin causes you to feel full earlier, causes your metabolic rate to increase, and stimulates your sympathetic nervous system. Unfortunately, the early fullness signal and the increased metabolic rate die off, and what you are left with is the sympathetic stimulation. But what is the cause of increased fat?

It is a positive calorie balance. That means that you eat more calories in your food than you burn in exercise and daily life. But what is the cause of increased calories? It is an increase in calorie-dense food. Some foods have more calories in them than others. For instance, if you want 200 calories of butter, you only get one tablespoon. But if you want 200 calories of celery, you have to eat over 3 pounds of it! So, if you eat more foods that are high in fat or sugar, you will have high calorie-dense food that will give you more calories before you feel full. But what is the cause of an increase in calorie-dense foods in your diet?

It is your taste. So, what is the cause of your taste? It is developed over time by repetitive choices. In other words, it is developed by habit. But what is the cause of your habits?

It has to do with your appetites. But what is the cause of your appetite? It is the result of your human nature. But what is the cause of your human nature?

It is sin. Ultimately, if we take any disease and go through this same process of asking ourselves the question, "what is the cause of this, and what is the cause of that?" and so on, we will always come to the same conclusion: sin. If it were not for sin, there would be no disease. What I don't want you to think is that I believe that it is always your sin that causes your disease. We know with Job that he was a righteous man, and yet the enemy was permitted to torment him with a terrible disease. It was still the result of sin, though. It was the enemy's sin that caused Job's disease.

Sin & Disease

What is sin? Sin is breaking the law. John tells us, "...for sin is the transgression of the law."[1] What law is this talking about? It is God's law, also known as the 10 commandments. But what is the

---

[1] 1 John 3:4 KJV

foundation of God's law? The foundation of God's law is His character, which is founded on love.

Matthew tells us, "'You shall love the Lord your God with all your heart, with all your soul, and with all your mind.' This is the first and great commandment. And the second is like it: 'You shall love your neighbor as yourself.' On these two commandments hang all the Law and the Prophets."[2]

You see, the foundation of His law is love.

And we read that "The law given upon Sinai was the enunciation of the principle of love, a revelation to earth of the law of heaven."[3]

We find, then, that disease, in many cases, is the result of a love problem.

"There is a divinely appointed connection between sin and disease. No physician can practice for a month without seeing this illustrated...If he will be observing and honest, he cannot help acknowledging that sin and disease bear to each other the relationship of cause and effect."[4]

This is so true. As a practicing physician, I cannot but help see that there is a connection between people's disease and sin. It isn't so easy helping them see the relationship, however. But it helps to be able to reason from cause to effect.

The Law of Cause & Effect

We can reason from cause to effect because there is a law of cause and effect that governs the association between causes and their effects. The law of cause and effect can be simply understood. Every effect must have a cause, and every cause must produce an effect. The cause always comes before or at the time the effect is produced, and the effect always comes after or at the time of the cause. If the

---

[2] Matthew 22:37-40
[3] White, E. G. (1896) *Thoughts from the Mount of Blessing*. (p 46). Mountain View, CA: Pacific Press Publishing Association.
[4] White, E. G. (1923) *Counsels on Health*. (p 325). Mountain View, CA: Pacific Press Publishing Association.

effect is present, the cause or its secondary causes must also be present, because if the cause, or its secondary causes, is removed, the effect must cease.

"The will of God establishes the connection between cause and its effects. Fearful consequences are attached to the least violation of God's law. All will seek to avoid the result, but will not labor to avoid the cause which produced the effect. The cause is wrong, the effect right...."[5]

You see, the effect is never wrong. It is a natural consequence of law. It is the cause which is wrong, and which must be sought out, identified, and removed. It is pointless to deal with the effect only, because the effect is not the problem, the cause is. Treating symptoms, in the long run, does no one any lasting good. We must search for the cause and remove it, then the effect will cease. The cause is wrong, the effect right.

When we consider the law of cause and effect, we find a reason why it functions the way it does. That explanation comes from one of the laws of thermodynamics. That law states that "All energy necessary for a system to function must come from outside of that system." Because of this, you cannot produce a perpetual motion machine. There is no machine that you can put in motion that will run indefinitely, generating all the power that it needs to continue to function. This is because it is always dependent upon energy from outside of itself to continue to function.

Since all energy necessary for a system to function (and all energy necessary for a system to dysfunction) must come from outside of itself, the effect cannot create itself. Because of that, the cause must be sought for from outside of the system in question. So, if someone has cancer in the left breast, one shouldn't go to the cancer in the left breast to find the cause. The energy necessary to cause the dysfunction had to come from outside of there.

---

[5] White, E. G. (1864) *An Appeal to Mothers*. (p 26). Battle Creek, MI: Seventh-day Adventist Publishing Association.

Laws of Function

Now, there is a law of function as well. And that law says that everything that functions is governed by unchangeable laws. For instance, human beings have a healthy blood salt or sodium level of 135-145 mEq/dL. It doesn't matter if you are from Australia, Africa, Antarctica, or America, all human beings have a blood sodium that ranges near 135-145 if you are healthy. But if it goes too low or too high, you cannot remain healthy.

Also, blood pH for human beings is 7.35-7.45 no matter where you are on the planet. So, if you think you would be better off with an alkaline blood pH of 8.5 and you achieve your goal, you will be dead, because the law that governs the function of the blood pH level in human beings determines that health is maintained between a pH of 7.35 and 7.45. If you like it or not, if you know about it or not, it doesn't matter. The law is what the law is, and you can't change it just because you like it or don't like it.

Similarly, body temperature (oral temperature) is somewhere around 98.6°F/37°C. There is a slight variation amongst people, but no one can live with a body temperature of 50°F, and no one can live with a body temperature of 150°F. It doesn't matter if you are tall or short, skinny or fat, black or white or blue. The law is what the law is, and you can't change it. Functional laws do not change. If we move to the arctic, we can't just choose to live by a freezing body temperature. And if we eat lots of salt, we can't just decide to live by a higher sodium level. We function how we function because of laws that govern our function, and those laws are not subject to change.

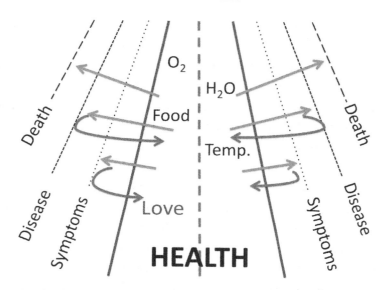

The Highway of Health

We are talking about The Law of Life, and to begin illustrating this law, let us consider the highway of health. Imagine with me for a moment that we have a road with two ditches on either side of the road. Health is maintained if you stay on the road, but if you veer off into either ditch, you will have problems. To begin with, we must define some of the things we need in order to maintain health. What are some of those health needs that we have?

One is oxygen. What else? Water too. What else? Nutrients, or food, is needed as well. But what else? We also need a certain amount of warmth to be healthy.

What happens if your temperature goes up? You have a fever. And how do you feel when you have a fever? Do you feel comfortable or uncomfortable? You feel uncomfortable. You develop symptoms. Those symptoms help you to know that you are outside of the confines of the law of body temperature, and your response to these symptoms, like sweating, being flushed, moving to the shade, turning on a fan, etc. help your body to return back to a lower temperature so that you can be back in the confines of the law that governs the function of your body temperature.

But what about the opposite direction? What if your temperature goes down? You get symptoms there too. Symptoms like goose bumps and shivering. Are these symptoms comfortable, or uncomfortable? Uncomfortable. Why? To let you know that you have deviated from the law.

You see, you and I don't really care about the law. We care about how we feel. If we stay on the road, it promotes comfort, which we enjoy. If we get off the road, it is associated with discomfort, to let us know that something is wrong and that we need to do something about it. These uncomfortable symptoms are part of your attempt to return your body temperature to normal so that you can be healthy again. It is returning you to the law by which you function so that you can function properly and feel better.

What would happen if you felt the same way when your temperature went up and when it went down? For example, if your temperature goes up, you feel hot. But if your temperature goes down, you feel hot also. That would be dangerous, because you wouldn't know what to do to get back into conformity with the law of your body temperature. If your temperature was going down and you felt hot, you would do everything to make your temperature go down faster, and you would quickly die. It is a good thing that it "hurts" differently when you deviate from the law one way than it does when you deviate from the law the other way. Because of this, you know what to do to get your temperature back to normal.

But what if you deviate further from the law than just symptoms? Let's say that your temperature goes up a lot. Instead of you just having symptoms, you develop disease (dysfunction), like heat exhaustion or heat stroke.

Now you feel really bad. Why? Because you are really in trouble. You are farther away from the law that governs the function of your body temperature. But the disease, even though it is more severe, is itself an effort to get your attention so that you can get your temperature down and back into line with the law that governs your body temperature. The same is true in the opposite direction. If you get really cold, you may develop disease, like frost bite, or chilblains, or hypothermia. This too, although more severe, is an effort to get you back into line with the laws by which you function so that you can experience health and comfort again.

Now if you don't stop at symptoms, and you don't stop at disease (dysfunction), if you continue to deviate farther and farther from the laws by which you operate, you will eventually go from dysfunction to no function (death). The body can only handle so much before it must give up.

And the same is true in the opposite direction. If the body temperature continues dropping, you will eventually die from hypothermia and abnormal heart rhythms. As we stay on the pathway, it is usually comfortable. As we deviate from the pathway, it becomes more and more uncomfortable, in order to let us know something is wrong so that we can do something about it and come back into the confines of the law that governs your function.

As you deviate away from the law toward death, you eventually cross a boundary called the point of no return. You are still alive, but you aren't going to get back to normal. Hopefully, before crossing this boundary, you cross the "pride line." The pride line is the line where your symptoms are bad enough that you will accept or ask for help in recovering from your discomfort and dysfunction.

From my medical experience, I have observed that women reach the pride line sooner than men. This is why women will typically seek medical attention sooner than men will. Sometimes, a man's pride line is so close to death that they will reach the point of no return before they will ever seek for help. This is unfortunate, to say the least.

Another factor that we can consider is this. If all of the other things that you need (oxygen, water, and nutrients) are all within the confines of the laws that govern their function, then when you deviate from the law of body temperature, you can go further from the pathway before you develop dysfunction and death. You can handle more of a deviation in one area if all the other areas are okay. But, if you are dehydrated, you have low oxygen levels, and your electrolytes are all messed up, your body temperature can't go up or down much before dysfunction and death.

Let us, for a moment, consider medication or other forms of symptom management in relation to this Highway of Health. If the manifestation of pain and discomfort (negative symptoms) are for the purpose of letting you know something is wrong and for motivating you to do something about it to return to the confines of the law that governs your function and which protects your comfort and proper function, what is the danger of pain medication or other forms of symptom care that do not address the underlying problem?

Let us say that you deviate from the law and you develop pain as a consequence. If you take pain medication, it decreases the intensity of the pain, therefore decreasing your motivation to do something about your problem. If you take increasingly stronger medication to mask your increasing pain, you blunt your motivation to do something about your situation and continue to drift closer and closer to death without the proper motivation to earnestly do something about removing the cause.

This is not to say that pain medication in an acute situation (trauma, surgery, etc.) is inappropriate. But symptom care in the long term counteracts the very motivations that have been put in place to help us comply with the laws that govern our being and make us more apathetic about remaining in a state of dysfunction and discomfort.

Now, I would like to ask you a question. How many of you need love? Of thousands of people that I have asked this question of, I have yet to find one person who does not need love.

We all need love, just like we need oxygen, water, nutrients, and warmth. Is it possible that there is a law that governs the function of love, and that if we deviate from that law, in either direction, that we will develop uncomfortable symptoms, then disease (dysfunction), and then eventually death? I propose to you that this is indeed the case. And as we discussed earlier, the law that governs the function of love is God's law—the ten commandments. We will see later how that law governs the function of love.

So, in this law of life, we find that health is proper function because the laws that govern our function are followed. Conversely, disease is dysfunction because we have in one way or another broken the laws which govern our function.

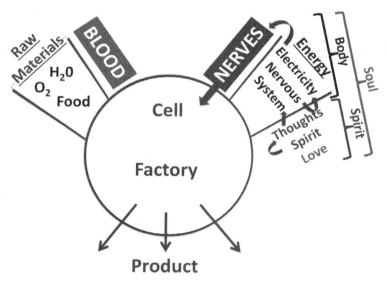

Cellular Factories

How many cells in your body need oxygen? How many need water? How many need food? And how many need warmth? All of them do. And how many of your cells need the effects of love? Every cell in your body needs the effects of love. But how do we get to the cells that which they need?

Before we answer this, let us look at the cells and their function. The cells are the smallest units of life. It is as simple as you can get and still have all of the functions of life in one package. Your body is composed of 50-100 trillion cells, and the function of your body as a whole is dependent upon the proper function of each cell. If enough cells dysfunction, you begin to notice the dysfunction. And the fewer the number of cells there are for a particular function, the fewer of them can dysfunction before you feel the effects.

It is stated that one can lose up to half of the existing cells responsible for a particular function before one actually has noticeable symptoms related to the loss of that function. For example, if you had 2 billion beta islet cells, which are responsible for producing insulin, you would need to lose about 1 billion of them before you started developing diabetic symptoms.

This is an important concept to understand when considering the law of cause and effect. If there is an effect (diabetes), there has to be a cause in place. The cause came before the effect was produced. Once the cause is present, it starts producing its effect. But the effect might not be large enough to be noticed for quite a while. For example, if you have a cause that begins destroying beta islet cells one by one, you won't notice until you have lost about half of your cells. It is estimated that diabetes has been in the process of developing for at least 10 years before one begins to manifest diabetes. So, the cause can be in place for a long time before the effect is large enough to be noticeable.

The cells in your body are like factories—chemical factories. They produce chemical products. Their products may be hormones, like the leptin or insulin we talked about earlier. They may produce proteins, cell signaling molecules, and any number of other chemical products.

But for a factory to be able to produce a product, what must it have? It must have raw materials. What are the raw materials that a cell uses? It uses oxygen, water, and nutrient (which are all chemicals). So, the cell takes raw materials, which are chemicals, and converts them into products, which are chemicals. And how do you get all of these raw materials to all of the cells of the body? You get it to the cells through the blood.

This means that the circulation of blood is vitally important to your health. If there is anything that impedes the flow of blood to a cell, tissue, organ, or organ system, there will be dysfunction in that cell, tissue, organ, or organ system to the degree that the circulation is deficient in supplying the needed raw materials.

But if you have a factory with a blueprint, workers, and raw materials, you still can't make a product. What else do you need?

You need to have energy, or power, in order to function. You have to plug the factory in! Remember, all energy necessary for a system to function must come from outside of that system. In the cells, what form of energy do the cells ultimately function by? It is electricity.

The cells maintain a difference in charges across the cell membrane, with the inside of the cell being more negatively charged and the outside of the cell being more positively charged. Positively and negatively charged particles separated by an impermeable or selectively permeable membrane form a battery. So, your cells are like little batteries. And the difference in charge is called voltage. If the charged particles then flow from one side of the cell membrane to the other, that is called current. It is this electrical activity at the cell membrane that drives the functions in the cell, even driving the breakdown of glucose and other molecules and releasing chemical or heat energy.

But where do the cells of the body get the electrical stimulation from in order to function and be coordinated with other cells in their function? It comes from the nervous system. Every function in the body is regulated through the central nervous system. All

21

mechanisms that maintain a balance of function in the body (called homeostasis) are regulated through the central nervous system.

The brain generates electrical energy that is transmitted down the nerves to the various parts of the body to stimulate the cells to function properly and to coordinate their function by increasing and decreasing their activity.

"The influence of the mind on the body, as well as of the body on the mind, should be emphasized. The electric power of the brain, promoted by mental activity, vitalizes the whole system, and is thus an invaluable aid in resisting disease."[6]

How does the energy from the nervous system get to all the cells of the body in order to control their function? It is transmitted down the nerves to the different parts of the body.

"The mind controls the whole man...Yet many spend all their lives without becoming intelligent in regard to the casket that contains this treasure. All the physical organs are the servants of the mind, and the nerves are the messengers that transmit its orders to every part of the body, guiding the motions of the living machinery."[7]

But where does the brain get the electricity that it generates and sends down the nerves to the rest of the body? Remember, all energy necessary for a system to function must come from outside that system. The energy that powers the brain comes from spiritual information, which, for simplicity's sake, I will call thoughts. Thoughts generate electrical activity in the cortex of the brain which is then transmitted down the nerves to the rest of the body.

Science claims that it is the electrical activity that causes the thinking, but it is actually the thinking that causes the electrical activity. Science believes that the electrical activity within the context of the neural networks of the brain produces thought. In other words,

---

[6] White, E.G. (1991) *Counsels for the Church* (p. 209). Nampa, ID: Pacific Press Publishing Association.

[7] White, E.G. (1897) *Special Testimonies on Education* (p. 33). Ellen G. White Estate, Inc.

science believes that the physical creates the spiritual. But we learn in the Bible that God (who is Spirit) created all that is. We find that it is the spiritual creates the physical, not the other way around. It is not the electrical activity within the context of the neural network of the brain that creates thought. It is thought, applied to the neural network of the brain that creates electricity.

The law of the conservation of energy states that energy is not lost, it is simply converted from one form to another. For example, the potential energy of a ball at the top of a hill is converted to kinetic energy when it begins to roll down the hill. The power of moving water, through a turbine, is converted to electricity. Nuclear power is converted to heat energy which is converted to electricity. The chemical energy of glucose is converted to cellular function and muscular movement in an animal. And the power of spiritual information (thought), when it strikes the physical structure of the brain, is converted to electrical energy that is then used to power and control the entire organism.

Thought is not physical. It is spiritual. And in order for you to bring to the body something that is spiritual, you need a part of you that is able to receive the spiritual and apply it to the body. And that part of you which is spiritual, which, combined with the physical structure of the brain, converts thought to electrical activity, is your spirit.

So, your spirit transmits spiritual information which is converted at the cortex of the brain into electrical impulses which are conducted down the nerves to each of the cells of the body so that they can be supplied with electrical impulses and their function can be controlled.

Remember, you and I need love. But do each of the cells of your body need love itself? No. They need the results (power, control, coordination) of love. The part of you that needs love is your spirit.

And if your spirit has the love (spiritual information) that it needs, it will produce the thoughts that are necessary to provide the energy and coordination necessary for the cells to function as they are supposed to. But if the spirit does not have the love that it needs, the energy and coordination will be messed up, and you will have dysfunction manifest in the body.

We were created in the image of God (Genesis 1:27), which means that we were created to think like God thinks. "God is love,"[8] and God's thoughts are thoughts of love. "For I know the thoughts that I think toward you, says the Lord, thoughts of peace and not of evil, to give you a future and a hope."[9] As we think like God thinks, it will promote the proper energy and coordination of the body's functions. But as our thinking deviates from God's thinking, it will cause dysfunction in the body.

So, in order for your cells to produce a good product, they need a proper blueprint for that product in the DNA, they need a proper environment in which to work, they need proper raw materials, and they need proper energy or control.

Causes of Dysfunction

So, what are some causes of dysfunction in the cells and therefore in the body?

One cause is <u>inheritance</u>. Inherited diseases are diseases that manifest in the individual as the result of changes in the genetic code of one's parents, grandparents, etc. and which manifest regardless of environmental or lifestyle factors in the individual. These include conditions like Huntington's chorea and cystic fibrosis—conditions which lead to disease and early death despite all attempts to cure it. Inherited causes of dysfunction are problematic, because you can't remove the cause, because the cause is in a prior generation. You can't remove the secondary cause (which is the change in the DNA

---

[8] 1 John 4:8
[9] Jeremiah 29:11

sequence), because the secondary cause is in every cell of your body, and we don't have a way of fixing the DNA in all of your cells. You can try to help with the manifestations of the disease, but you cannot remove the disease, because you can't get to the cause. This, however, doesn't mean that God can't remove the cause. He is not limited by time. He can recreate anew.

This definition is different than saying that a condition is genetic. Many diseases in one way or another are genetic, because in order for you to manifest that disease, you must dysregulate or mutate proper genes, or you must express improper genes.

Another cause of dysfunction is <u>environment</u>. The cells function within the context of certain environmental parameters. You can cause dysfunction because of too much or too little pressure. You can be hit by a car, shot by a gun, stabbed by a knife, or have dysfunction because of a SCUBA diving accident. All of these involve too much pressure that causes damage to the cells. You can also have damage because of too little pressure (vacuum injuries, high-altitude illness, etc.). You need a certain amount of environmental pressure in order for your cells to function, and when the pressure is too low, dysfunction is the result. Also, if the temperature surrounding the cell is too hot or too cold, it cannot function properly, even though it has the proper raw materials and energy. You can burn your fingers or freeze your toes and cause dysfunction.

Finally, we are surrounded by electromagnetic waves in various forms, and the intensity and frequency of those waves can cause damage. To get a severe sunburn from ultraviolet waves, or to have significant radiation exposure from x-ray devices or nuclear spills or nuclear bombs can damage many cells in the body. So, pressure, temperature and electromagnetic radiation are environmental issues that can impact function or dysfunction.

Another potential cause of dysfunction is <u>raw materials</u>. You may have harmful raw materials, things like toxins, poisons, envenomations, etc. You may simply have the wrong materials—soft drinks instead of water, fried foods instead of fruits, and nitrogen instead of oxygen. You may have an imbalance of the proper raw materials. You may have too much salt, too little carbohydrates, too much fat, and so on.

If the cause of the dysfunction is because of raw materials, the effect will eventually be generalized. Certain cells or tissues may require certain raw materials more than other cells do, so the manifestation of the dysfunction may begin locally (for example, hypothyroidism caused by low iodine levels, death of the brain before death of the toes in drowning, etc.), but as the cause continues or worsens, all the cells will eventually be involved as a cascade of metabolic consequences spread throughout the other cells of the body.

But dysfunction may be caused by <u>energy</u> as well. Unlike raw materials issues, energy issues typically cause local dysfunction initially. Remember, the cells function by electrical energy, and that electrical energy is stimulated and coordinated by the nervous system, and the brain generates that electrical energy by thinking. The nervous system is very specific. One area of the brain controls or receives information from one place in the body, and another spot on the brain does the same for another place in the body. If you have a particular electrical problem in one part of the brain, it can be transmitted down the nerves to particular parts of the body to affect that specific location. So, if you have a local problem, it can't be caused by just raw materials.

For instance, some people have problems with gout. Gout is a painful inflammation of a joint (sometimes several joints) because a substance called uric acid forms crystals in the joint and causes irritation, pain, redness, swelling, and heat. Most individuals with gout have elevated levels of uric acid in their blood, and when you draw their blood from their arm, the uric acid levels are high. So, we assume that the cause of the problem is the uric acid, and we give medication to lower the uric acid level and the gout goes away. But is gout caused by uric acid only? Where did you get the blood from that showed the elevated uric acid levels? The arm or the hand. Because of the law of diffusion, we know that dissolved substances in water distribute themselves evenly throughout the water so that the concentration is the same throughout. So, we know that when we measure uric acid levels in the arm, the uric acid level in the blood in the toe is nearly the same. The uric acid is elevated throughout the body, so why does it cause a problem just in the one joint? If it is just caused by the uric acid, it can't. There must be something else. The uric acid must only be a cofactor.

I suspect that it is an energy issue from the nervous system that is the primary problem. The uric acid is only a cofactor that is necessary in order for the problem to manifest itself. It is the same thing with cholesterol and arterial plaques/blockages. How is that the case, you ask?

The concentration of cholesterol in the blood just before a cholesterol plaque is essentially the same as at the plaque and after the plaque. So, what caused the cholesterol to accumulate in one spot here and another spot there and create a 90% blockage here and a 75% blockage there? It couldn't just be the concentration of the cholesterol. There had to be something else to cause the accumulation of the cholesterol.

We know that inflammation is essential to the process of plaque formation, but what causes the inflammation? Science assumes that it is local trauma caused by abnormal blood flow at the area of the artery where the plaque develops, but I suspect that it is the signals sent to that particular area of the artery by a specific nerve which originated as a thought in a specific part of the cortex of the brain.

What do we know about the connection between the thoughts and the function or dysfunction of the body? One series of experiments were conducted between 2000 and 2013. The investigators were studying a chemical to see if it could be used as an anti-inflammatory medication. As part of the process of testing the chemical for human use, they needed to run many animals through various tests first.

One of the tests was injecting the chemical into the fluid space that surrounds the brain (called an intrathecal injection). This is to discover what would happen if the substance was able to get across the blood-brain barrier. What the investigators found out was that when they performed the injection, the mice stopped producing tumor necrosis factor alpha (TNFα), a prominent inflammatory chemical in the immune response.

The confusing aspect of this response was that TNFα is not produced in any significant degree in the brain. After a number of years, the investigators discovered that when the chemical was injected around the brain, it changed the signal that was being sent down the vagus nerve to the spleen. In the spleen, that signal was received by the T-helper cells (part of the immune system), and the T-helper cells communicated with the natural killer cells (other cells in the immune system which are predominantly responsible for producing TNFα), and the natural killer cells turned off their production of TNFα.

The investigators wanted to know if they could cause the same result without the chemical, and they eventually were able to stimulate the vagus nerve with an electrical nerve stimulator and produce the same result! This opened up many possibilities of treating various problems in the body by manipulating the signals received through the nerves.

Recent research also shows that there is a strong connection between the nervous system and cancer. Studies have shown that the

28

nervous system can influence every step in cancer development, growth, and spread, promoting or limiting the metastasis of cancer. And how do you and I control this every day of our lives? By our thoughts and attitudes! Perhaps this is why we see so many people who develop cancer within months to several years of a major stressor or loss in their life. Perhaps this is why we see so many individuals who eat a plant-based diet and exercise regularly, but who still develop and die from cancer.

Finally, dysfunctions can be caused by the Enemy. We see this in the life history of Job. He was a righteous man, faithful in all he did, but the enemy came to God and made a complaint of God being unfair—that Job would not serve God like he did if God stopped protecting him. So, God gave the enemy permission to cause dysfunction or disease in Job. It wasn't an inheritance issue, it wasn't an environment issue, it wasn't a raw materials issue, nor an energy issue. It was a direct attack of the enemy. The same can be true today as well. Unlike Job, however, many times the Enemy has access to us because we give him that access by participating with him in sin.

CHAPTER TWO

Learning from My Needs

Basic Needs		Delivery Pathway			Action	Make
Raw Materials	Oxygen	Lungs	→	**BLOOD**	Breathe	No
	Water	Stomach	→		Drink	No
	Food	Stomach	→		Eat	No
	Warmth	Skin	→		Expose/ Cover	No
	Sunshine	Eyes/Skin	→		Open/ Expose	No
	Sleep	Brain	→		Close eyes	No
Energy	Love	Spirit	→	**NERVES**	Think	No

Basic Needs

L et us look at our basic needs again, but from a slightly different angle.

There are basic needs that the cells have in order to function, including raw materials and energy. The raw materials include oxygen, water, nutrients, and warmth, as we have already pointed out. But it also includes sunshine and sleep.

And in order for these basic needs to get to the cells of the body, they first need to get into the body through an organ or organ system. We have to have a way of getting the basic need from where it is to where it needs to go—we need a delivery pathway.

So, what organ or organ system is responsible for bringing into the body the oxygen that you and I need in order to live? The lungs.

And what organ or organ system is necessary for us to bring into the body the water that we need in order to live? The stomach.

And what organ or organ system is necessary for us to bring into the body the nutrients that we need in order to live? The stomach as well.

And what organ or organ system is necessary for us to bring into the body the warmth that we need in order to live? The skin.

And what organ or organ system is necessary for us to bring into the body the sunshine that we need in order to live? The eyes and the skin.

And what organ or organ system is necessary for us to bring into the body the sleep that we need in order to live? The brain.

As we have noted earlier, once these raw materials are brought into the body by their respective organs or organ systems, they then need to be delivered to all of the cells of the body so that the cells can life.

And what is responsible for distributing the raw materials to the cells? The blood.

And what is responsible for distributing the power or electricity to the cells so that they can live? The nerves.

Now, we must consider the fact that not only do we require certain basic needs, and not only do we need a delivery pathway to get those needs to the cells, but there is also an action that is required to bring those basic needs into the body. So, what action do the lungs need to perform to bring into the body the oxygen that you need in order to live? The lungs must breathe.

And what action does the stomach need to perform to bring into the body the water that you need in order to live? The stomach (which represents the digestive tract) must drink.

And what action does the stomach need to perform to bring into the body the food that you need in order to live? The stomach must eat.

And what action does the skin need to perform to bring into the body the warmth that you need in order to live? The skin must expose or cover itself.

And what action do the eyes and skin need to perform to bring into the body the sunlight that you need in order to live? The eyes must open, and the skin must expose itself.

And what action does the brain need to perform to bring into the body the sleep that you need in order to live? The brain must close your eyes, lie down, etc.

For every basic need there must be an action that an organ or organ system performs in order to bring the needed substance into the body, and then it must be distributed to each of the cells. But there is something else that we all need, which we have discussed previously.

We all need love. But what action is necessary to bring the love that we need into the body? That action is thinking. It is by thinking that love is converted to proper energy and brought into the body, transmitted down the nerves, and carried to the cells of the body.

Let us consider love a little closer. How much does love weigh? How many protons, neutrons, and electrons is it made of? That's ridiculous, you say! Love is not physical, is it? So, in order to bring love, which is not physical, into the body, we must have an organ that is itself not physical. So, what is that organ? It is the spirit. The spirit, which is not physical, is the organ that brings love into the body through the action of thinking, which is then transmitted by the nervous system, through the nerves, to every part of the body.

Now, we must ask ourselves a very important question. Can you create the oxygen that your lungs need to breathe in order for you to live? No. You can use chemicals or machines and extract the oxygen from other molecules and concentrate oxygen into a container, but you cannot create oxygen from nothing.

Similarly, can you create the water your stomach needs to drink in order for you to live? No.

And can you create the nutrients that your stomach needs to eat in order for you to live? No. You can participate in the growing process by planting, watering, weeding, etc., but you cannot give the seed life and make it grow and produce.

Can you create the warmth that your skin needs to cover or expose itself from/to in order for you to live? No.

And can you create the sunshine that your eyes need to open to, or your skin needs to expose itself to in order to live? No.

Can you create the sleep that your brain needs to prepare for in order to live? Anyone who has experienced insomnia will tell you, "No!"

And can you create the love that your spirit needs to think by in order for you to live? No. You cannot.

Action vs. Basic Need

Can we have health if we have the wrong substance, even though we have the right action? For example, when we breathe air with oxygen in it, we will maintain health. But if we breathe carbon monoxide, what will happen? It will kill us. The same action (breathing) with the wrong source (carbon monoxide) will bring death.

If we drink the water that our bodies need, we will maintain health. But if we drink antifreeze, it will kill us. The same action (drinking) with the wrong source (antifreeze) will bring death.

If we eat foods with proper nutrients, we will maintain health. But if we eat rat poison, it will kill us. The same action (eating) with the wrong source (rat poison) will bring death. If we think good thoughts, which are based upon love, we will maintain health. But if we think bad thoughts, it will kill us. The same action (thinking) with the wrong source (thoughts not consistent with love) will bring death.

Only if we have the right action (breathing, drinking, eating, thinking) with the right source (O_2, H_2O, good food, love) can we expect health. If we have the right source (proper nutrients, O_2, etc.) but the wrong action, (overeating, hyperventilating, not eating, not breathing, etc.), that will lead to disease and death. If we have the right action (breathing, drinking, or eating), but the wrong source (poisons, toxins, etc.), that will lead to disease & death. And if we have the wrong action (overeating) and the wrong source (poison), it will lead to disease & death.

What My Needs Tell Me

When we seriously think about the various needs that we have, we learn something about ourselves. Can you create that which you need? No. If you could, it wouldn't be a need of yours. The body cannot create that which it needs. And the spirit cannot create that which it needs.

Do you need love? Yes! Absolutely! Then, can we create or produce love? No! If we could, it wouldn't be a need of ours. Now, is this an individual problem? It is just you and I that cannot produce love, or is this true of all humanity? It is a human problem, not just our problem. No human being can create or produce love. We need to remember this, because this is foundational to many of our problems.

Can someone else breathe for me? No. I must breathe for myself. Only the oxygen that I breathe will benefit my body. Can someone else drink for me? No. Can someone else eat for me? No. Only my actions—not the actions of another—affect my health.

Another human being cannot be the source of that which I, as a human being, need, because they need that very thing as well. So, let me ask this question. Can another person be my source of love? No! Because they are in need of it themselves.

Basis of Relationship Issues

Suppose that you have a neighbor that comes over all the time to borrow something from you. Then one day, she comes over and tells you that her daughter has a rare lethal health condition that can only be treated in a special center in Russia, and it will cost $5,000,000 for treatment. Because it is Russia, payment is required in full before beginning treatment. She asks you for all of the $5,000,000 so they can get treatment. You politely tell her that you don't have the money, but you give her a donation toward their goal.

But each day she comes back and keep asking for the rest of the $5,000,000. Eventually, what do you do when she comes to your house and knocks on your door? You don't answer the door!

You are frustrated because you don't have what she needs, and she is frustrated because she isn't getting what she needs. This is how it is in relationships. We get frustrated when others don't give us the love we need, and they get frustrated because they can't give it to us. We expect from others what is impossible for them to produce. The problem is that we are going to the wrong source!

Whose Responsibility?

Whose responsibility is it for me to be filled with oxygen? It's my responsibility. And whose responsibility is it for me to be filled with water? It's mine. And whose responsibility is it for me to be filled with proper nutrients? It's mine.

Have you ever, for any period of time, felt less than 100% full when it comes to love? I have a question for you. Whose responsibility is it for me to be filled with love? Is it God's responsibility or is it mine? It is my responsibility! You see, if it were God's responsibility, we are told that "He does all things well." How well does He do all things? Perfectly well. And how often does He do all things well? All the time. So, if you have ever, even once, felt less than 100% full of love, that, in and of itself, is evidence that it is not God's responsibility to fill you with love. It is your responsibility to take the love you need. It is His responsibility to make sure that love is available.

Years ago, a group of people killed themselves by their own action of breathing. They were taken to a gas chamber, and their action of breathing killed them, because they breathed the wrong substance. But they had no choice. The environment was chosen for them, and as it was the wrong one, and they died.

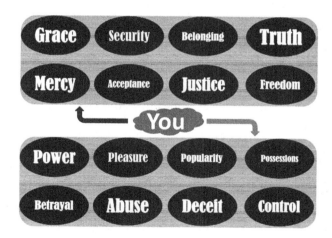

The Buffet

Imagine that you have been fasting for several days, and it is time to break your fast. You go to a buffet restaurant in town that is known for having tasty, but healthy, options. You grab your tray, plate, bowl, spoon, fork, knife, and napkin and wander through the restaurant looking at the various options to see what you are going to eat this time and what you are going to skip. But you do something curious. You leave your tray, plate, bowl, spoon, fork, knife, and napkin behind and leave the restaurant. And you are still hungry.

Whose fault is it that you are still hungry? It is your own fault. It isn't the restaurant's responsibility to feed you. It is their responsibility to make sure the food is available and that it meets certain standards, but it isn't their responsibility to feed you. It is your responsibility to take the food you want and eat it.

God has a buffet. His buffet involves things like grace, security, belonging, truth, mercy, acceptance, justice, and freedom. These are all different aspects of love. As I go through the restaurant, I have the opportunity of filling my plate with, and subsequently eating, each of the options available, but I don't have to. I could walk through the restaurant, smell the wonderful smells and see the beautiful sights, and never take a single item. It is God's responsibility to provide the buffet of love, but it is my responsibility to take from it and make it mine.

But there are some aspects of God's buffet of love that are different from a regular restaurant. God's buffet of love is always stocked. It is never empty. It is always open. It is never closed. It is always what I need. It is never unhealthy. And God has paid for it all so that it's free.

God tells us, "I will never leave you nor forsake you."[10] "I have loved you with an everlasting love; therefore with lovingkindness I have drawn you."[11] "Ho! Everyone who thirsts, come to the waters; and you who have no money, come, buy and eat. Yes, come, buy wine and milk without money and without price."[12] We can never be where God's buffet of love is not available to us, so we can never be in a situation where we don't have access to the correct source for our healthy thinking.

---

[10] Hebrews 13:5
[11] Jeremiah 31:3
[12] Isaiah 55:1

But God's buffet is not the only buffet available. Everyone else has a buffet that they offer to you as well. But since others are in the same situation of selfishness as we are, they offer buffets of selfishness. These buffets offer dishes like power, pleasure, popularity, and possessions. But they also offer dishes like betrayal, abuse, deceit and control.

It is said, "You are what you eat." When you eat an apple, the components of the apple are broken down and assimilated so that they become a part of your body. Similarly, when we eat from the buffet of others, we assimilate what they have, and it becomes a part of our mind.

Have you ever noticed that when someone close to you gets upset, you get upset? Or when they are happy you get happy? Or if they are depressed, you get depressed? It is because we are eating from their buffet and we become like them. But we don't have to eat from their buffet.

You see, others may provide a hurtful buffet for you, but just because they do so, it doesn't mean that God's buffet of love all of a sudden disappeared. His buffet of love is always available, no matter who or what is around you and what kind of buffet they are offering.

It is your choice whether you will take from God's buffet of love, or whether you will take from "their" buffet of selfishness. And what buffet you choose to take from determines your outcome.

But before you start beating yourself up, remember, human nature naturally takes from the buffets of selfishness. We naturally feed there. And many persons do not realize that there is a buffet of God's love and that it is available to them all the time. So, we have, almost by default, taken from others' buffets.

But now that you know, you can begin to take from the right buffet. What is it that allows you to take from the one buffet or the other? It is faith/belief/trust. The one you believe or trust in, you will take from. The one you do not believe or do not trust in, you will not take from. So, taking from God's buffet of love necessitates trusting and believing Him. We will cover this more fully later in this book.

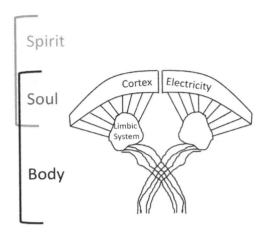

The Body & The Spirit

Now, let us take a different look at how we are made and how we function. This is a simple drawing of your brain. The cortex is on the surface of the brain and the limbic system is deeper down in the brain. The cortex is where thinking, reasoning, and other higher brain functions occur. It directs the "work" of the nervous system. It produces electricity that is then transmitted down the wires (the nerves) to the various parts of the lower brain and body.

We can see this electrical activity when we do an EEG. The different leads that are placed on the scalp pick up the electrical activity that is generated and transmitted below it in the cortex, and we can study the pattern of electrical impulses to determine if there are particular problems going on in the brain.

The limbic system, which resides deeper in the brain, below the cortex, is primarily involved in emotions, the control of the fight or flight response, and assisting with memory. The cortex and the limbic system then connect with the rest of the body through the wires, the axons or the nerves.

The brain and the rest of our physical being that it is connected to is the body. But are we only physical? When man was created in the first place, there were a few components that were put together to make him. We read in Genesis 2:7, "And the Lord God formed man of the dust of the ground, and breathed into his nostrils the breath of life; and man became a living being." So, God took dust, and added to it his breath, and the combination of the two became a living being. The dust corresponded to the body. The breath corresponds to the spirit. And the living being corresponds to the soul. It's like God married the body and the spirit together at creation.

In Genesis we read, "Therefore a man shall leave his father and mother and be joined to his wife, and they shall become one flesh."[13]

Synergism

When a man marries a woman, the combination of the two is not numeric. It is synergistic. Numeric is one plus one equals two. Synergistic is one plus one equals nine. You see, as individuals, a man and a woman cannot reproduce. But as a couple, they can. In our family, we have 6 children, so in our case, $1 + 1 = 8$. The total is greater than the sum of the parts. This is synergism.

Conflict

Similarly, the breath and the dust are synergistic, forming a soul that is more than the sum of the body and the spirit. But the soul still involves both the body and the spirit.

How many of you like conflict? What is conflict anyway? Conflict is defined as a "Strong disagreement between people, groups, etc., that results often in angry argument." Can you have conflict in just one thing? No! Have you ever had a conflict with yourself? How can you have a conflict if you are just one? Don't you need at least two to have a conflict? Are you just one? No. We are physical AND we are spiritual.

Our body includes the brain and the rest of the body. It is the part that senses and interacts with the physical world around and within us. The spirit is different. It is the part of us that communicates life to our physical being, or imparts spiritual power, which is necessary for the physical being to function. The soul, however, is not

---

[13] Genesis 2:24

a third entity. It is the synergistic union of the physical and the spiritual. The soul is conscious and aware. It is what thinks and reasons, interprets and understands. The soul is where the spiritual power unites with the physical body, enabling us to be living, thinking beings. In us, the soul is located in the brain.

You can cut off your finger, and you are still you. You can cut off your arm, and you are still you. You can cut off your leg and you are still you. You can even cut out your heart and replace it with someone else's heart, and you are still you. But you cannot cut off your head and still be you. That is where the soul is located.

Different Needs

Are your physical needs and your spiritual needs the same? Your physical needs include oxygen, water, nutrients, warmth, sleep, and sunshine. But your spiritual needs include grace, harmony, security, belonging, acceptance, liberty, righteousness, truth, and understanding. All of these spiritual needs are different components of love.

So, which needs are greater, your spirit's needs, or your body's needs? To answer this question, we simply need to look at one example—fasting.

When you are fasting, what is your body "saying"? It is saying, "Give me food." And what is your spirit saying back? "No!" Your physical needs include food, but your spiritual needs include freedom (from disease, pain, suffering, social oppression, etc.), or a deeper relationship with God (by fasting, which helps the mind to become clearer and better able to listen to the Holy Spirit). When the body sends a signal up to the cortex, is it a command or a request? Does the spirit have to comply with the information sent to it by the body? No. The spirit has the choice. But when the spirit sends a signal to the body, is it a request or a command? It is a command. The body cannot decide to not do what the spirit tells it to do.

As we see in the example of fasting, your spiritual needs—the need of love—is greater than your physical needs. The spirit is in charge.

CHAPTER THREE

Deceptions of Love

The Gift

T hink about the person in the world that you love the most. Imagine that there is a special event coming up (birthday, anniversary, etc.), and you want to surprise them with something that they will really like. You put thought and time into finding just the right gift. You spend your hard-earned money on the gift, and you wrap it so nicely for them. When the time comes, you bring the gift to their house, knock on the door, and they open the door, take the gift, throw it on the ground, stomp on it, and walk back inside, slamming the door shut. How do you feel? Why do you feel that way?

Let's look at another scenario. This time, you need some extra money, so you get a job with UPS. You get your route and stop at one of the locations for a delivery. You grab the package, take it to the house, knock on the door. The person comes to the door, signs your little signature thingy, takes the package, throws it on the floor, stomps on it, and goes back inside and slams the door shut. How do you feel? Why do you feel that way? What is the difference between scenario one and scenario two?

In the first scenario, the reason that I am hurt is because I think, "It's mine." It's my present that I gave. It was my money that the present was purchased with. It represents my love. And that was my person (spouse/friend/parent/child/etc.). Whereas, in the second scenario, it's not mine. It's not my present. It's not my money. It doesn't represent my love. And it's not my person.

If I think it's mine, I am personally hurt (hurt for myself) when it is rejected. If I don't think it's mine, I'm not personally hurt if it is rejected. But beyond that, when I give, I have expectations. I, as a human being, give in order to receive back again. And in the first scenario, I am hurt because I didn't receive back what I expected.

You see, human love gives to receive. It is an investment. An investment is putting something of value in something with the expectation of gaining a greater return. You have heard the phrase, "No strings attached", right? In humanity, there's no such thing. There are always strings attached. As human beings, we give with expectations of return. And our expectations determine how much return is necessary in order for us to be satisfied with our investment.

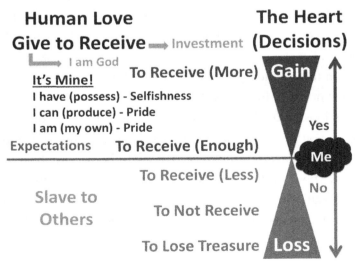

The Heart - Human

The heart that we will be talking about is not your blood-pumping muscle. The heart is the center of the mind where decisions (subconscious decisions) are made. You and I make decisions based upon only two criteria. All decisions that we make in the heart emerge from these two criteria. One criteria upon which decisions are based is gain, and the other criteria upon which decisions are based is loss. And you and I are created in such a way that we always respond with "yes" to gain, and we always respond with "no" to loss.

It is a little more complicated than that. You see, we choose between various losses and gains. We will choose a greater gain above a lesser gain. And we will choose a smaller loss above a greater loss. And the weight of what is considered a gain and loss and how great that gain or loss is considered is based upon our value system, or treasures. The Bible tells us, "Where your treasure is, there your heart will be also."[14] God designed us to always win, to always gain, to always grow in positive experiences. Heaven will be a continual gaining, learning, growing, improving. Throughout eternity we will gain more and more.

Because we are created to always choose yes to gain and no to loss, the enemy cannot tempt us to lose. It is no temptation at all to us. If I have a cup that has something that looks like water, but is actually full of mercury, strychnine, arsenic, and other poisons that will surely kill you; if you know it is poisonous and will kill you, are you tempted to take it and drink it? No, it is no temptation at all. The enemy couldn't come to Eve with the forbidden fruit and say, "Here, eat this; you'll die." That would be no temptation at all. What he had to do was trick her into believing that loss was gain and gain was loss.

You see, in the Garden of Eden, God told Adam and Eve, if you eat of the fruit of the tree of the knowledge of good and evil, you will lose (you will die). But if you don't eat it, you will gain (you will live).

[14] Matthew 6:21

45

Genesis chapter 3 tells us the story, "Now the serpent was more cunning than any beast of the field which the Lord God had made. And he said to the woman, 'Has God indeed said, 'You shall not eat of every tree of the garden'?' And the woman said to the serpent, 'We may eat the fruit of the trees of the garden; but of the fruit of the tree which is in the midst of the garden, God has said, 'You shall not eat it, nor shall you touch it, lest you die." Then the serpent said to the woman, 'You will not surely die. For God knows that in the day you eat of it your eyes will be opened, and you will be like God, knowing good and evil.'"[15]

The enemy told Eve the exact opposite of what God had told her. He probably added that he had been eating from the tree for months or years and that he hadn't died, and in fact, he had even gained the ability to talk. "Nothing bad will happen to you, Eve. In fact, you will be better off than you now are if you eat the fruit, because you will be like God."

God said, if you eat it, you lose. The enemy said, if you eat it, you gain. God said, if you don't it eat, you gain. The enemy said, if you don't eat it, you lose. And what did Eve do?

"So when the woman saw that the tree was good for food, that it was pleasant to the eyes, and a tree desirable to make one wise, she took of its fruit and ate."[16] Eve was deceived. She believed the lie of the enemy, and once she was convicted that to eat was gain, she ate it. Why? Because she was created to always say yes to gain.

The enemy promised Eve that if she ate of the forbidden fruit, she would be like God. Could it be that you and I believe the same lie today?

In the human heart, we harbor certain expectations, and these expectations are intricately tied to the love by which we function.

Love, in a sinful, fallen, human context, gives to receive. We give to others with an expectation of return. This love is an

[15] Genesis 3:1-5
[16] Genesis 3:6

investment. We put something of value into someone else so that we can get something of greater value back. We may give roses, or teddy bears, or poems, but we are looking for acceptance, belonging, and harmony. And if I give in order to receive, then my gain is to receive. But how much do I need to receive in order to be satisfied, in order to be in gain? I will consider myself to be in great gain if I receive in greater quantity something similar to that which I gave (two hugs in return for one given), or if I receive something different than that which I gave, but which is of greater value to me than that which was given (acceptance or belonging in exchange for a rose). But I am also in gain if I receive at least enough in return from my investment. If I receive, but I receive less than I expected to receive, I perceive that I am in loss. And if I don't receive anything at all in return for my investment, I am in even greater loss. Also, if my treasure is taken away (my house burns down, my car is stolen, my spouse leaves me for someone else, my child dies, etc.), I am at loss as well.

If I have high expectations, I will be at loss more often. But if I lower my expectations, I won't lose so much because it is easier for them to meet my expectations. In human love, I have to lower my expectations in order to limit my losses.

Let us consider a young couple. One day the young man passes the young woman, and there is an attraction. He sees her, interacts with her, and begins to think, "She is a gain." But he's not sure, because gain is receiving, so he gives her something to see if he'll get something back. He gives her a smile, time, and conversation, and she returns the favor. Gain! He was giving (investing), and she was receiving, so that was a gain to her. So, he invests a little more and a little more, and she does the same in return. Both are happy because both are gaining, because both are receiving. Both continue to raise each other's expectations by sharing letters, flowers, teddy bears, time, interest, companionship, etc.

Eventually, the young man is sure that she is a permanent gain, but he's not sure if she thinks he is a permanent gain. Finally, he "pops the question," and asks her to marry him. She, having received so much from him, believes he is a permanent gain as well, and says yes. Life continues this way until one day...they get married! Then, he has to go to work. He remembers that he had hobbies before he met her, like sports, fishing, etc., and he remembers that he has other friends as well. So, letters and flowers and teddy bears come less and less often. She now has only one way to mitigate her losses—she must lower her expectations. If she doesn't lower her expectations, she will be at loss, and the heart always says, "no" to loss.

So, over time, he gives less and less and less, and she has to lower her expectations more and more and more in order to remain in gain. But eventually she says, "Enough is enough," and she doesn't lower her expectations any more. If he continues to perform below her expectations, she will continue to be at loss, and the heart always says no to loss, so she will eventually either look for another gain, or "cut her losses" and separate or divorce.

This is how the human heart functions, and this is why we see so many marriages end in divorce. It all has to do with gain and loss.

The problem with human love, the reason that we feel personally hurt, is that we think it's mine. And "it's mine" has several components to it. I have—meaning it is my possession. It belongs to me. I can—meaning I produced it. It came from me. And I am—meaning I am my own individual being, answerable to myself, responsible for the production and the use of the thing in question.

From a love standpoint, I believe that I possess love, because I produced the love, because I am my own self, capable of creating love from myself so that I can give it away. But let me ask you this, how much of what you possess is actually yours? We are told, "'The silver is Mine, and the gold is Mine,' says the Lord of hosts."[17] Does that include the gold and silver in your bank account? Yes, it does. It is all His. How much did you create? Nothing. So, can you lay claim to anything as your own? No. He is the Creator, therefore everything is His. Everything we have is the Lord's. He is the One who possesses. We are only the stewards.

But when I think things are mine, when I think they came from me, and when I think that I am my own, I take it personally when my gift is rejected. I am hurt when I am not recognized and not appreciated, and when the gift is rejected. Why? Because it's about me—it's mine.

If you have two children playing in a playground and there is a toy dump truck that they are playing with that belongs to the one boy, and the other boy takes the truck and starts playing with it as if it belongs to him, not sharing with the boy who owns it, we say that the boy who took the toy is selfish. To treat things (including love) as if it is your possession, when in reality it belongs to God, is selfishness. 1 Corinthians 4:7 tells us, "And what do you have that you did not receive? Now if you did indeed receive it, why do you boast as if you had not received it?" Don't treat God's possessions as if they are your own. They are His, not yours.

What character quality underlies the thought that I can produce/create/make anything on my own and that I am my own person to do whatever I want to with myself? It is pride. So, we find in the core of our human heart that we are selfish and proud. In fact, selfishness and pride are the only motivations that the sinful, fallen human heart can come up with for everything that it does. Human love—giving to receive—is always motivated by selfishness and pride, and it always has expectations relative to self. I have expectations for myself and what I will receive in return for what I invested.

---

[17] Haggai 2:8

Don't be mistaken. Selfishness can give. Pride can sacrifice. But it does so with the objective of receiving greater rewards in return. The love that I have for my loved ones (spouse, children, parents, friends, pets, etc.) is a selfish love. You and I cannot come up with anything different. At the core of who we are, we find selfishness and pride.

God tells us the truth about ourselves in the Bible when He says, "But we are all like an unclean thing, And all our righteousnesses are like filthy rags; We all fade as a leaf, And our iniquities, like the wind, have taken us away."[18] We have nothing good in ourselves. Our righteousness is like menstrual cloths. That is all we have to offer. So, when we offer God the gift of our heart, we aren't offering anything of great value. We are offering trash. But God is happy when we offer Him our hearts, because He can then come in and recreate us in His image and instill within us that which *is* of value.

I want to be painfully clear about something right now. This is the human heart, and this is how it functions in every sinful human being that has ever lived since the fall. The best that you and I have; the best we can do; the love we have for our children, parents, spouses, friends, or others; the motivation behind all of the good that we do; the gifts that we give; or the sacrifices that we make; all are motivated by selfishness and pride. That is it. There is nothing else. There is nothing better than selfishness and pride as motivations in the sinful, human heart.

But that is not all. It gets worse! Can you give what you do not have? No. You must take something from someone or somewhere else first in order to have something to give. Who, in all the universe, can give first without first taking? Only God. So, when I give first in order to receive back, I put myself in the place of God. I think I am God, thinking that I possess or produced "it" in the first place so that

---

[18] Isaiah 64:6

I can give it away in order to get something back again. I am living by the lie that the enemy told Eve in the garden, "you will be like God." So, when you and I give to receive, what we are revealing is that we believe that, "I am God." I have the capacity of God to create the love, which I then give away, in order that I may receive more love in return. This heart is motivated by selfishness and pride and puts me in the place of God. And this here is always breaking the first commandment. "You shall have no other gods before Me."[19]

What is the most common God we have before God, that thing which causes us to break the first commandment on a daily basis? It is self. I am number one in my life. My wants, my desires, my wishes, my needs come first. God comes somewhere down the line.

And this heart—which believes it is God, which is motivated by selfishness and pride, whose gain is receiving, and loss is not receiving, not receiving enough, or having my treasure taken away—this heart is a slave to others. You see, my gain or loss is dependent upon whether "they" give or not and how much they give. And I can't control them. I can't make them give, but I am dependent upon what they give in order to be in gain. And I can't control whether they reject me, leave me, or die. I am a slave to others, because I am dependent upon them and what they give me in order to be in gain. And because you must control a source that you do not trust, and because no human is completely trustworthy, you and I always attempt to control others so that we can control our gains and losses.

We may try to control them with the good (praise, thanks, gifts, etc., in order to receive similar things in return), or we may try to control with the bad (coercion, guilt trips, shame, accusation, abuse, etc.) in order to force them to remain as our source and to continue to give to us. But whether it is with the good or with the bad, we try to control others, because they are our source, and we can't trust them. We are slaves to others.

---

[19] Exodus 20:3

The Heart - Deceived

We've been talking about the heart and how it functions from a human love standpoint. But I want to know how do I know if Christ is in my heart? Let's read. "How am I to know that Christ is in my heart? If, when you are criticised or corrected in your way, and things do not go just as you think they ought to go,—if then you let your passion arise instead of bearing the correction and being patient and kind, Christ is not abiding in the heart."[20]

Ouch! Is it possible that this is true? Then what about you and me? Where do we stand? How can we be in such a miserable position when we thought we were at least somewhat okay? It is because... "The heart is deceitful above all things, and desperately wicked; who can know it?"[21]

What does it mean that the heart is deceitful above all things and desperately wicked? It means that the human heart is crazy. It is crazier than anything else out there.

I don't know if you have ever met someone who is crazy. In my medical school rotations, I did inpatient and outpatient psychiatric rotations, where I met individuals who had very interesting alternate realities. I met many more when I was studying and practicing as an emergency physician.

Some patients would believe that a microchip was implanted in their brain, and the military was sending them signals through that microchip and causing them to do things. Others had voices that spoke to them and demanded that they do certain things. Others believed that they had super powers and could walk through walls. Others believed that the news anchor was speaking to them directly through the TV and giving them secret messages that only they understood.

After taking care of many individuals who had significant alternate realities, I came to understand one thing. I couldn't talk

---

[20] White, E. G. Union with God. *Review & Herald*, July 12, 1887, paragraph 9.
[21] Jeremiah 17:9

anyone out of their alternate reality. They were as convinced that their alternate reality was real as I was convinced that my reality was real. The only thing that would wake them up to see a different reality was a strong medication.

Could it be the same for you and me? What if we were all crazy? What if all of us had the same delusional state and believed the same alternate reality? How would we know we were sane or crazy? If everyone we checked with believed essentially the same thing that we did, and we were all wrong, how would we know?

What God is trying to tell us is that we are crazy. The core of who we are—our heart—is crazy! And it is crazy in a particular direction. It is crazy for wickedness. It is like having a ball on the side of a smooth hill. When you let the ball go, it will always roll downhill. It will never roll uphill. No matter how many times you try, it will always roll downhill. Downhill is wickedness. Uphill is righteousness.

Not only does the human heart always go downhill toward wickedness, if unrestrained, it will always go to the deep end of the wickedness pool. Why is that? Imagine that you are born into a world that is upside down. It has always been upside down, and since it has always been upside down, it appears to you to be right side up. God has created you with a desire to gain, achieve, grow, learn, improve, etc. You see a mountain in the distance, and you want to climb to the top of it, so you do. But what happens if you are upside down? The higher you climb, the lower you go, thinking that you are pursing greatness, you climb to the lowest depths that you can go. This is the craziness/deception of the human heart and why it always goes to the deep end of the wickedness pool.

What does it mean to be desperately wicked? It means to be desperate for wickedness. Imagine being in a desert. You have been there for a couple days without any water, and you are dying. Your lips are cracked and bleeding. Your tongue is dry and sticking to the roof of your mouth. You have a pounding headache and you feel fatigued and dizzy. And off in the distance you see a table, and on the table is a glass pitcher of water, glistening in the sunshine, revealing the ice cubes inside.

Now, imagine that between you and the water is a cactus patch. Would you brave the cactus patch in order to get the water? Yes, you would. Why? Because you are desperate for the water. That is how the human heart relates to wickedness. It is desperate for it!

You and I have an amazing capacity to be deceived. We don't know what is in our hearts. We don't understand ourselves. We can see fairly clearly what is wrong with others, but as far as we are concerned, we are blind.

We see this clearly pointed out by Jesus in the sermon on the mount. He says, "And why do you look at the speck in your brother's eye, but do not consider the plank in your own eye? Or how can you say to your brother, 'Let me remove the speck from your eye'; and look, a plank is in your own eye? Hypocrite! First remove the plank from your own eye, and then you will see clearly to remove the speck from your brother's eye."[22]

We can see a speck of a problem in our neighbor, but we can have a 2x4 sticking out of our head and not have a clue about what is going on. How can this be? Let me illustrate with an example.

When I first purchased glasses, they were very awkward. They sat on my nose, hurt the tops of my ears, and made everything look a bit distorted. I didn't like them, but I needed to see, so I put up with them. One day, I couldn't find my glasses. I was looking all over the place for them and couldn't find them in any of the usual locations. Eventually, I asked my wife to help me find my glasses. She looked straight at me and said, "Honey, you're wearing them!" How embarrassing! Here I was, looking all over the place for my glasses, and the whole time they were right there on my face. I had become

---

[22] Matthew 7:3-5

so accustomed to them that my mind ignored all of the signs of their presence.

In fact, just the other day our family was having evening worship together, and one of the girls was missing. I was looking around the room to see where she was. The others noticed that I was puzzled, so they asked what I was looking for. I told them, and they all started laughing! The missing child was sitting in my lap!

You and I have lived with ourselves for so long, that there is a lot about us that we don't notice. When was the last time that you noticed your eyelashes in your vision? They are always there, always in the way of your peripheral (and sometime central) vision. But do you notice them? No. Why? Because they have been a part of you for so long, you ignore their presence (until they fall out and get in your eye!). We have serious character flaws, but we just don't see them. If we were born with a 2X4 handing out of our head, we would become so familiar with it, that we would stop noticing it (until we hit something with it).

Is it possible that our ability to be deceived is so great that even God could look us in the eye, tell us what is wrong with us, and we wouldn't believe Him? If you said no, are you so sure? Are you better than Jesus' disciples?

In Mark 8:29, Peter and the disciples claim that Jesus is the Christ—the Messiah—and just two weeks later, that same Jesus looks at Peter and the disciples and says, "'All of you will be made to stumble because of Me this night, for it is written: I will strike the Shepherd, and the sheep will be scattered....' [Did they believe Him?] Peter said to Him, 'Even if all are made to stumble, yet I will not be.' Jesus [the same Jesus who they had just affirmed was God] said to him, 'Assuredly, I say to you that today, even this night, before the rooster crows twice, you will deny Me three times.' [God is looking Peter and the disciples in the eyes and telling them what is wrong with them, and do they believe Him?] But he [Peter] spoke more vehemently, 'If I have to die with You, I will not deny You!' And they all said likewise."[23]

Even if God looked you in the eye and told you what was wrong with you, you probably wouldn't believe Him. You see, we are crazy, and you can't convince someone that they are crazy just by telling them that they are crazy. You need powerful medication to wake them up to see that they are crazy. In life, that medication is called demonstration.

We are deceived. So, what is the solution? We need God to show us what is going on by demonstration. You and I don't know our hearts. But someone does. Jeremiah 17:10 goes on to say, "I, the Lord, search the heart, I test the mind, even to give every man according to his ways, according to the fruit of his doings."

God knows what is in our hearts, and we must come to Him to reveal to us (demonstrate) what is there.

David, the man after God's own heart, may have faintly understood that there was something in his heart when he prayed the this prayer in Psalm 139:23 & 24, "Search me, O God, and know my heart; try me, and know my anxieties; and see if there is any wicked way in me, and lead me in the way everlasting." If God would have looked at David in the eye and told him that he was a lust-driven murderer, David probably would have argued with God.

"Surely not Lord. I delight to do Your will, O my God, and Your law is within my heart.[24] I will set nothing wicked before my eyes; I hate the work of those who fall away; it shall not cling to me."[25]

But David, in Psalm 139, asks the lord to "try me." It is in the trial that we discover what is in the heart.

One day, David was walking around his palace, when he saw a lovely woman bathing on her roof. Maybe he said, "Whoa" quickly and thought about walking away. But he took a double take,

[23] Mark 14:27-31
[24] Psalm 40:8
[25] Psalm 101:3

"Whooaa!" Then he asked someone what her name was. Then he invited her over. And one thing led to another, and one year later David had committed adultery with Bathsheba, had murdered her husband, had a baby with her, and was fast heading to complete ruin. Then enters the prophet Nathan with a story of a rich man who has many sheep and a poor man who only has one sheep and loves it and even shares his home with it. A stranger comes to the rich man, and the rich man, sparing his own flock, takes the poor man's sheep and slaughters it to feed the stranger. David, in his anger, calls down curses upon the rich man in the story, and then Nathan points at David and tells him, "You are the man!"[26] At that point, because of the trial and the prophet's words, David's eyes are opened, and he sees what is in his heart. It isn't good at all! He now knows that he needs something.

Now, we find David praying another prayer about the heart, "Create in me a clean heart, O God, and renew a steadfast spirit within me. Do not cast me away from Your presence, and do not take Your Holy Spirit from me. Restore to me the joy of Your salvation, and uphold me by Your generous Spirit."[27] David now knows, without a doubt, that he needs a new heart.

When God allows the trial to come to us, and in the trial what is inside of us spills out and reveals to us what is in our heart, we then realize that we desperately need a new heart. And when we, like David, knowing that we need a new heart, come to God and plead for that new heart, God answers us.

"I will give you a new heart and put a new spirit within you; I will take the heart of stone out of your flesh and give you a heart of flesh. I will put My Spirit within you and cause you to walk in My statutes, and you will keep My judgments and do them."[28] God knows what the human heart looks like. He knows how horrible it is. He knows all

---

[26] 2 Samuel 12:7
[27] Psalm 51:10-12
[28] Ezekiel 36:26,27

about the selfishness and pride and putting ourselves in the place of God. He knows! And He knows that we need a new heart, so He died so that He could give us a new heart—His heart. Do you want that heart today?

"Lord, I see how bad my heart is. I see that everything is motivated by selfishness and pride. I have nothing, absolutely nothing, to offer you. But I need a new heart—your heart. Would you give me that new heart, and put Your Spirit within me? Thank you, Jesus, for doing that for me; not because I deserve it, but because You love me. Amen."

CHAPTER FOUR

The Law of Life: Take to Give

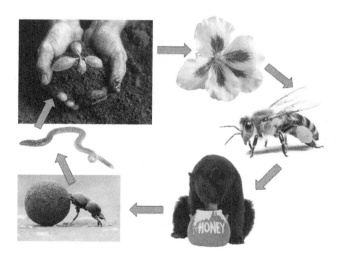

Give or Take?

Now, when it comes to love, can I give first, or do I have to take first? Can you give what you don't have? No. We must take first in order to have something to give. Otherwise, we are God, producing and possessing that which we give. This is true throughout all creation.

Does a seed that is planted in the ground first give to the ground, that it may grow, or does it first take from the ground that it may grow? It takes first. It takes of the moisture and temperature and nutrients, and as it grows and breaks through the ground, it takes of the sunshine. It takes and grows and takes and grows.

Suppose that the seed in question produced an orange tree. For whom does the tree produce the fruit? For itself? No. It has no personal gain from the fruit which it produces. Can other orange trees benefit from what it produces (other than other trees growing from the seeds)? No. It takes from what is in the ground so that it can give to other species. Even the oranges that land on the ground do not immediately benefit the tree. Those oranges must first "give" to bacteria or fungus or other creatures, which eventually give to the ground, which can then give to the tree.

The seed takes from the ground so that it can produce a flower so that it can give the pollen to the bee. The bee takes of the pollen so that it can give honey to the bear. The bear takes of the honey so that it can give to the dung beetle. The dung beetle takes of the dung so that it can give to the worm. And the worm takes of what was provided so that it can give back to the soil.

We see this Law of Life—this circuit of beneficence—exemplified in the life of Christ. "Looking unto Jesus we see that it is the glory of our God to give. "I do nothing of Myself..." "I seek not Mine own glory," but the glory of Him that sent Me...In these words is set forth the great principle which is <u>the law of life</u> for the universe. All things Christ received from God, but <u>He took to give</u>. So in the heavenly courts, in His ministry for all created beings: through the beloved Son, the Father's life flows out to all; through the Son it returns, in praise and joyous service, a tide of love, to the great Source of all.

And thus through Christ the circuit of beneficence is complete, representing the character of the great Giver, the law of life."[29]

Just like the circuit of life, the circuit of beneficence, taking to give, is the law of life.

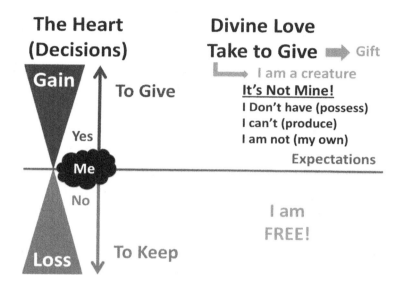

The Heart – Divine

God wants to give us a new heart. He didn't design for us to have the old heart of human love. He intended for us to operate by divine love. And divine love does not give to receive, it is the Law of Life—taking to give. Instead of investing in others, looking for a return from what I give, divine love gives without an expectation (for myself) of return. I still have expectations, but my expectations are for your benefit, not for me.

I expect my wife to love me, because I know that if she does, that means that she is connected to God. He is in control of her life, and that connection brings her life, love, joy, and peace. So, for her sake, I expect her to love me. But I don't have that expectation for

---

[29] White, E. G. (1898). *The Desire of Ages.* (p 21). Mountain View, CA: Pacific Press Publishing Association.

myself. I don't need her to love me for my own sake, because she is not my source. God is my source, and I take all I need from Him, and then I give it away to my wife and others.

I will never run out of love because I am connected to the source which does not run out, and as I take that love and am filled by it, I have all that I need to give away to other without ever going empty.

And if I take in order to give, then my gain is to give. And If my gain is to give, then my loss is to keep it to myself.

This follows a divine law outlined in John 12:25, "He who loves his life will lose it, and he who hates his life in this world will keep it for eternal life." What Jesus is showing us here is that in reality, if you want to keep something, you have to give it away, because the moment you hold on to it and try to keep it to yourself, you lose it.

So, if you need acceptance, go to God and take it from Him. He has all the acceptance you need, for He is the source of it. But it you want acceptance to remain yours, you must give it away to others—you must accept them. If you need belonging, go to God and take belonging from Him. He has all the belonging you need, for He is the source of it. But if you want belonging to remain yours, you must give it away to others—you must let them belong. If you need forgiveness, go to God and take of His forgiveness. He has all the forgiveness you need, for He is the source of it. But if you want forgiveness to remain your own, you must give it away to others—you must forgive them.

So, what about God? Can He keep His love to Himself? Or must He give it away? He must give it away! It is His very nature to give. If He kept it to Himself, He would lose, and God doesn't lose. He always wins, so He always gives. We are told, "He makes His sun rise on the evil and on the good, and sends rain on the just and on the unjust."[30] His giving is not about you, it is about Him and His character, for it is a reflection of His heart.

And the same is true for you and me when Christ lives in our hearts by faith. Our reward is secured by giving. "...the law of self-sacrifice is the law of self-preservation. The husbandman preserves his grain by casting it away. So, in human life, to give is to live. The life that will be preserved is the life that is freely given in service to God and man. Those who for Christ's sake sacrifice their life in this world will keep it unto life eternal."[31]

This heart of divine love remembers, "It's not mine." I don't have, or possess, it. It simply doesn't belong to me. It belongs to God. I can't produce anything. I'm not a creator. Only God is. So, whatever I have comes from Him—even my creativity.

And I am not my own to do whatever I want with myself. I am not my own, because I was bought at a price.[32] I belong to God and I am responsible to Him. And just like the UPS delivery guy, if the gift is rejected or destroyed or not appreciated, it doesn't affect me personally, because it's not mine and it doesn't represent me. I'm not personally hurt by others response to my love, because I am not dependent upon them—I am dependent upon God—and what they do with the gift is their problem (a reflection of their own heart), not mine. And besides, it wasn't my gift anyway. It came from God.

The Example - Jesus

Let us take Jesus as our example. Did he believe that He possessed anything of His own? No. He said, "Foxes have holes and birds of the air have nests, but the Son of Man has nowhere to lay His head."[33] He recognized that everything that He had was from His father. He didn't possess anything.

---

[30] Matthew 5:45
[31] White, EG. (1898). *The Desire of Ages.* (p 623). Mountain View, CA: Pacific Press Publishing Association.
[32] 1 Corinthians 6:19,20
[33] Matthew 8:20

Did Jesus believe that He could do a whole lot on His own? No. He said, "I can of Myself do nothing."[34] He recognized that all of His power and capabilities came from His Father.

Did Jesus believe that He was His own person, that He had the right to do whatever He wanted with Himself? No. He recognized, just like Paul did, that we are not our own. "Or do you not know that your body is the temple of the Holy Spirit who is in you, whom you have from God, and you are not your own? For you were bought at a price; therefore glorify God in your body and in your spirit, which are God's."[35]

So, Jesus didn't possess, didn't produce, and wasn't His own. Jesus was the ultimate UPS delivery guy. Was He selfish? Did He think about Himself, or was He focused on others? We are told, "Not for Himself, but for others, He lived and thought and prayed."[36]

If Jesus was convicted that He was just the delivery guy, if He was convicted that nothing was His, that all that He could do was from His Father, and that He was not even His own, then what could hurt him personally? Nothing! To be personally hurt is to think about self—to focus on what they did and what it means to me or did to me. Jesus didn't think of Himself. His concern was for others.

In John chapter 6, when Jesus was talking about Himself being the bread of life, and many of His followers left, and never followed Him again, was He hurt for Himself, or did He hurt for them? He hurt for them and what their decision meant to them. When Judas betrayed Jesus with a kiss, did He hurt for Himself because He was being betrayed by His friend? No. He hurt for Judas and what that betrayal meant to Judas. And when Peter denied Him with cursing to the servant girl, did Jesus hurt for Himself, or for Peter and what Peter's denial meant to him? Jesus hurt for Peter, not for himself.

---

[34] John 5:30
[35] 1 Corinthians 6:19,20
[36] White, E. G. (1900). *Christ's Object Lessons.* (p 139). Review and Herald Publishing Association.

Don't misunderstand me. Jesus did hurt. He was the man of sorrows and acquainted with grief. But His hurt was not for Himself, it was for others. His hurt for us was in proportion to His love for us, and since He loved infinitely more than we can love, he hurt infinitely more than we can hurt.

In His childhood, "Jesus did not contend for His rights. Often His work was made unnecessarily severe because He was willing and uncomplaining. Yet He did not fail nor become discouraged. He lived above these difficulties, as if in the light of God's countenance. He did not retaliate when roughly used, but bore insult patiently."[37]

As He grew into an adult and entered into the scenes of His ministry, we find that, "In the heart of Christ, where reigned perfect harmony with God, there was perfect peace. He was never elated by applause, nor dejected by censure or disappointment. Amid the greatest opposition and the most cruel treatment, He was still of good courage."[38]

"The Saviour's life on earth, though lived in the midst of conflict, was a life of peace. While angry enemies were constantly pursuing Him, He said, 'He that sent Me is with Me: the Father hath not left Me alone; for I do always those things that please Him.'" John 8:29. No storm of human or satanic wrath could disturb the calm of that perfect communion with God."[39]

And as He came to the end of His life and the weight of sin began to be laid upon His shoulders, His concern was not for himself. "He was now in the shadow of the cross, and the pain was torturing His heart. He knew that He would be deserted in the hour of His betrayal. He knew that by the most humiliating process to which criminals were subjected He would be put to death. He knew the ingratitude and cruelty of those He had come to save. He knew how great the sacrifice

[37] White, E. G. (1900) *The Desire of Ages*. (p 89). Review and Herald Publishing Association.
[38] White, E. G. (1898) *The Desire of Ages*. (p 330). Review and Herald Publishing Association.
[39] White, E. G. (1896) *Thoughts from the Mount of Blessing*. (p 15). Mountain View, CA: Pacific Press Publishing Association.

that He must make, and for how many it would be in vain. Knowing all that was before Him, He might naturally have been overwhelmed with the thought of His own humiliation and suffering. But He looked upon the twelve, who had been with Him as His own, and who, after His shame and sorrow and painful usage were over, would be left to struggle in the world. His thoughts of what He Himself must suffer were ever connected with His disciples. He did not think of Himself. His care for them was uppermost in His mind."[40]

How did He always respond to problems? "Christ never murmured, never uttered discontent, displeasure, or resentment. He was never disheartened, discouraged, ruffled, or fretted. He was patient, calm, and self-possessed under the most exciting and trying circumstances. All His works were performed with a quiet dignity and ease, whatever commotion was around Him. Applause did not elate Him. He feared not the threats of His enemies. He moved amid the world of excitement, of violence and crime, as the sun moves above the clouds. Human passions and commotions and trials were beneath Him. He sailed like the sun above them all. Yet He was not indifferent to the woes of men. His heart was ever touched with the sufferings and necessities of His brethren, as though He Himself was the one afflicted. He had a calm inward joy, a peace which was serene. His will was ever swallowed up in the will of His Father. Not My will but Thine be done, was heard from His pale and quivering lips."[41]

Even in His trial, He maintained His calm trust in His father. "One of his officers, filled with wrath as he saw Annas silenced, struck Jesus on the face, saying, 'Answerest Thou the high priest so?' Christ calmly replied, 'If I have spoken evil, bear witness of the evil: but if well, why smitest thou Me?' He spoke no burning words of

[40] White, E. G. (1898) *The Desire of Ages*. (p 643). Review and Herald Publishing Association.
[41] White, E. G. (1990) *Manuscript Releases Volume Three*. (p 427). Silver Spring, MD: Ellen G. White Estate, Inc.

retaliation. His calm answer came from a heart sinless, patient, and gentle, that would not be provoked."[42]

And when Peter denied Him with cursing, for whom was Jesus hurt? "While the degrading oaths were fresh upon Peter's lips, and the shrill crowing of the cock was still ringing in his ears, the Saviour turned from the frowning judges, and looked full upon His poor disciple. At the same time Peter's eyes were drawn to his Master. In that gentle countenance he read deep pity and sorrow, but there was no anger there. –The sight of that pale, suffering face, those quivering lips, that look of compassion and forgiveness, pierced his heart like an arrow."[43]

And what was His response when He was under the most intense physical suffering? "While the soldiers were doing their fearful work, Jesus prayed for His enemies, 'Father, forgive them; for they know not what they do.' His mind passed from His own suffering to the sin of His persecutors, and the terrible retribution that would be theirs. No curses were called down upon the soldiers who were handling Him so roughly. No vengeance was invoked upon the priests and rulers, who were gloating over the accomplishment of their purpose. Christ pitied them in their ignorance and guilt. He breathed only a plea for their forgiveness,—'for they know not what they do.'"[44]

What amazing love for those who hated Him! He never had a negative thought or emotion toward them!

The depth of His love is not just amazing to us. It was amazing to the angels. "With amazement the angels beheld the infinite love of

---

[42] White, E. G. (1898) *The Desire of Ages.* (p 700). Review and Herald Publishing Association.
[43] White, E. G. (1898) *The Desire of Ages.* (p 712-713). Review and Herald Publishing Association.
[44] White, E. G. (1898) *The Desire of Ages.* (p 744). Review and Herald Publishing Association.

Jesus, who, suffering the most intense agony of mind and body, thought only of others, and encouraged the penitent soul to believe."[45]

"Though calumny and persecution were heaped upon Him from the cradle to the grave, they called forth from Him only the expression of forgiving love."[46] This is what the new heart, operating with divine love, looks like.

Did He Suffer?

Did Jesus escape life without any suffering? No! He did suffer. "For it was fitting for Him, for whom are all things and by whom are all things, in bringing many sons to glory, to make the captain of their salvation perfect through sufferings."[47] Jesus was perfected through suffering. But who did He suffer for? "That those whom He had undertaken to save, those whom He loved so much, should unite in the plots of Satan, this pierced His soul."[48] He hurt for them, not for Himself.

Jesus, like us, shared humanity, and humanity longs for belonging, understanding, and companionship. Jesus shared that longing with us. "The human heart longs for sympathy in suffering. This longing Christ felt to the very depths of His being."[49]

"...a keener anguish rent the heart of Jesus; the blow that inflicted the deepest pain no enemy's hand could have dealt. While He was undergoing the mockery of an examination before Caiaphas, Christ had been denied by one of His own disciples."[50]

---

[45] White, E. G. (1898) *The Desire of Ages.* (p 752). Review and Herald Publishing Association.
[46] White, E. G. (1896) *Thoughts from the Mount of Blessing.* (p 71). Mountain View, CA: Pacific Press Publishing Association.
[47] Hebrews 2:10
[48] White, E. G. (1898) *The Desire of Ages.* (p 687). Review and Herald Publishing Association.
[49] White, E. G. (1898) *The Desire of Ages.* (p 687). Review and Herald Publishing Association.
[50] White, E. G. (1898) *The Desire of Ages.* (p 710). Review and Herald Publishing Association.

It is true that Jesus did not have a thought for Himself, and He did not hurt for Himself. But like us, Jesus hurt more for those who were closer to Him than those who were not. His ability to suffer was greater than our ability to suffer to the same degree that His ability to love was greater than our ability to love. His love for His children was so much greater than ours, that His suffering FOR them was so much greater than ours. And to the extent that we learn to love as He does, will be the extent to which we will be able to suffer as He did.

You see, "He is despised and rejected by men, a Man of sorrows and acquainted with grief. And we hid, as it were, our faces from Him; He was despised, and we did not esteem Him. Surely He has borne our griefs and carried our sorrows...."[51]

He was a man of sorrows and acquainted with grief, but it wasn't for Himself; it was for others!

What about Me?

This is Jesus. He was perfect. But what about you and me? How are we supposed to react in similar circumstances? "Christ did not fail, neither was He discouraged, and His followers are to manifest a faith of the same enduring nature....They are to despair of nothing, and to hope for everything."[52]

"If the works of the ambassadors of Christ are wrought in God, they will not be elated by praise from human lips; neither will they be depressed because they think they are not appreciated."[53]

"If you had the Spirit of Christ, you would not notice slights and make much of fancied injuries."[54]

"It is the love of self that destroys our peace. While self is all alive, we stand ready continually to guard it from mortification and

---

[51] Isaiah 53:3,4
[52] White, E. G. (1898) *The Desire of Ages*. (p 679). Review and Herald Publishing Association.
[53] White, E. G. (1888) In Demonstration of the Spirit. *The Review & Herald*. September 4, 1888, paragraph 3.
[54] White, E. G. Be Gentle Unto All Men. *The Review & Herald*. May 14, 1895, paragraph 4.

insult; but when we are dead, and our life is hid with Christ in God, we shall not take neglects or slights to heart. We shall be deaf to reproach and blind to scorn and insult."[55]

"A man whose heart is stayed upon God is just the same in the hour of his most afflicting trials and most discouraging surroundings as when he was in prosperity, when the light and favor of God seemed to be upon him. His words, his motives, his actions, may be misrepresented and falsified, but he does not mind it, because he has greater interests at stake. Like Moses, he endures as 'seeing Him who is invisible' (Hebrews 11:27); looking 'not at the things which are seen, but at the things which are not seen' (2 Corinthians 4:18). Christ is acquainted with all that is misunderstood and misrepresented by men. His children can afford to wait in calm patience and trust, no matter how much maligned and despised; for nothing is secret that shall not be made manifest, and those who honor God shall be honored by Him in the presence of men and angels."[56]

When God's love lives in us, the life of Christ lives out through us.

The Heart - Divine

This divine love, taking to give, gives us the key to entering into the life of Christ. Just like Jesus, I recognize that I am only a steward of God's resources. I must come and take from God first in order for me to have any love with which to love others. And the love that I give to others is a gift, not an investment. It comes without strings attached. It doesn't hurt me personally if they stomp on the gift and walk away. I don't hurt for myself, because I'm not thinking about myself. I hurt for them and am concerned about them.

---

[55] White, E. G. (1896) *Thoughts from the Mount of Blessing.* (p 16). Mountain View, CA: Pacific Press Publishing Association.
[56] White, E. G. (1896) *Thoughts from the Mount of Blessing.* (p 32). Mountain View, CA: Pacific Press Publishing Association.

And this heart, which understands that it is a creature and not God, is free! I am no longer dependent upon others. I no longer am dependent upon what others do and say in order to be in gain. My gain comes simply from giving, and I am the one who decides whether I give or not, so my gains and losses are under my control. I don't need to control others, because they are not my source. God is my source, and I don't need to control Him because I can trust Him. He is a faithful Source!

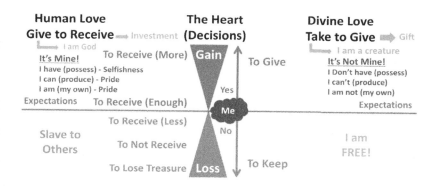

The other gains and losses of the fallen heart—receiving, not receiving, not receiving enough, or having it taken away—don't even enter into the equation of divine love in the new heart. My joy, my gain, my winning, is simply giving. This is divine love, and this love is impossible for you and me to produce. It, itself, is the gift of God, and we are dependent upon Him for it. We must come to God and take of His love—of the buffet of love that He has provided for each of us—so that it may be ours. To the degree that I am filled with this love is the degree to which I can share that love with others.

CHAPTER FIVE

A Decisive Treasure

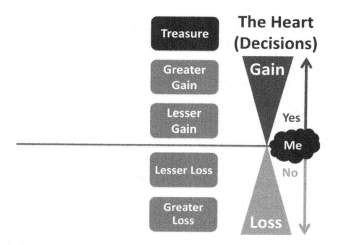

The Treasure

J esus tells us, "For where your treasure is, there your heart will be also."[57] What was He talking about? What is your treasure, and what does it have to do with your heart?

---

[57] Matthew 6:21

Your treasure is the system by which you and I determine how valuable something is, and whether that thing is a gain or a loss to us. And this valuation system is a function of the heart. Now that we have a good understanding of the heart and how it functions, let us focus in a little more on the treasure and the decision-making process.

If I give you the option to either receive $1,000 or to pay $1,000, which would you choose? You would choose to receive $1,000, of course. Why? It is because we always choose a gain over a loss.

Now, let us change the scenario a little. This time, you can either receive $1,000, or you can receive $10. Which would you choose? You would choose to receive $1,000. But why? It is because we always choose a greater gain over a smaller gain.

Let us try a third scenario. This time, you can choose whether you will pay me $1,000, or whether you will pay me $10. Which will you choose? You would choose to pay me $10. Why? It is because we always choose a smaller loss over a greater loss.

So, you see that we have a system by which we evaluate the relative value of something—whether it is a gain or a loss, and how valuable it is to us compared to other things. The magnitude of the gain is directly proportional to the value of the treasure being gained, while the magnitude of the loss is directly proportional to the value of the treasure being lost.

But in our hearts, value is not absolute. I assess the value of something based upon multiple criteria. There are several components that help to determine the relative value of the thing in question, and all of those factors come together to determine whether something is considered a gain, or whether it is considered a loss.

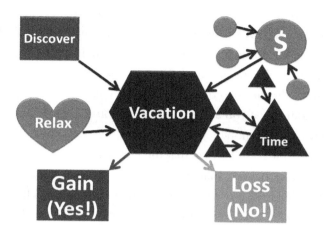

Let us take the decision to go on a vacation or not as an example. We might want to discover new sights and experiences. But it costs money to go, and I might miss out on income while gone. I would like to get away and relax a bit. But I only have a certain amount of time to finish the project that I am working on, and it is an important project.

If discovery and relaxation are greater gains to me than the loss of money and time, then I will choose yes to the vacation. But if they aren't, I will choose to not go on vacation.

If I have enough money in savings, if I have vacation time available so that I won't go without an income, and if I just received a bonus at work, that might change how I decide relative to the vacation. And if the project deadline gets put off, or someone else is added to the project so that it is not so dependent upon me, or I decide that my time is better spent on vacation than on the project, that also will influence whether I choose to go on vacation or choose not to go on vacation.

You see, our valuation system is not absolute. It is subjective. It is based upon our beliefs and convictions about the various variables involved in the decision-making process. But value is absolute. Value is objective. And true value is based upon God and His Word.

My perception of something's value can change by changing what I *believe* relative to that thing. And my perception of whether something is a gain or a loss can change by changing what I believe. And when the value or the status (gain vs. loss) of something changes, the decisions that are based upon that thing change accordingly.

For example, if you are living in a relationship with a spouse who is not giving you enough love, attention, respect, etc., you would naturally be in loss. Let us say that the concept of divorce enters your mind, and you believe that living in your current situation of not receiving enough love is a greater loss than divorce is. What will you do? Even though you consider divorce to be a loss, you will seek for a divorce. Why? Because you always choose a lesser loss over a greater loss, and you see divorce as a lesser loss.

But let us add another factor to the equation. Let us imagine that you read Malachi 2:16, "For the Lord God of Israel says that He hates divorce, For it covers one's garment with violence...." And, because you respect God and what He thinks, because God is a great gain to you, and his approval is important to you, divorce is now the greater loss, because it represents the loss of God's favor. If, because of this new information about God's hatred of divorce, you now view divorce as the greater loss, and your current situation of not being loved enough by your spouse as a lesser loss, what will you do? You will remain in the relationship of not receiving enough from your spouse, because by doing so you are avoiding the greater loss of divorce.

Remember, I can remain in a perceived loss only if by doing so I am avoiding a greater loss. And I can only do something that is perceived as a loss if I believe that by doing that thing, I avoid a greater loss.

Let us take another look at this decision-making process. This time, you are living in a relationship where your spouse is not giving you enough love, and you are in loss. But instead of considering divorce, you are now contemplating going out and finding another gain—another person to give you the love you are looking for. Divorce is a loss, but infidelity, in many ways, is a gain. It offers pleasure, attention, excitement, and so on. So, if you see your current relationship as a loss and you see infidelity as a gain, what will you do? You will choose infidelity over faithfulness to your spouse. You may "know" that it is wrong, but as long as you believe it is a gain (in your heart), you will always choose it over a loss (staying faithful to your spouse who is not loving you enough).

Now, let's consider this from a different perspective. Imagine that you are reading Revelation 2:22, "Indeed I will cast her into a sickbed, and those who commit adultery with her into great tribulation, unless they repent of their deeds," and you discover that God hates adultery. Because you love and respect God, you understand that, rather than being a gain, infidelity is a loss. And you believe that it is a greater loss than remaining faithful to the spouse who is not loving you enough. What will you do? You will choose to remain faithful to your spouse rather than be unfaithful.

So, when God is the greatest treasure of our life, when maintaining a connection with Him and retaining His favor is the top of our gain list, things change. Infidelity, which we once considered a gain, now, because we see that He hates adultery, it is no longer a gain. It becomes a loss.

Because God is the greatest treasure in our life, we no longer consider infidelity a gain, so it no longer is an option that our heart will choose. But what about divorce, which is a loss? When we have God as our greatest treasure and we understand that God hates divorce, it is no longer a greater gain than living with our spouse who isn't loving us enough, because participating in divorce would mean the loss of our greatest treasure—the favor of God.

So, because God is the greatest treasure of our heart, divorce and infidelity are losses to us. But not only that, since living with our spouse (who is not loving us enough) means that we are allowed to keep our greatest treasure (God's favor), then living with that spouse becomes a gain, because by doing so we can keep our greatest treasure. So, instead of believing that we are living in loss, we believe that we are in gain, because we retain our greatest treasure.

To stop doing something that we had perceived as a gain, we must: 1) adopt a greater gain in its place, or 2) believe it to be a loss by attaching it to a greater loss. This is where consequences come into the equation.

Let us imagine for a moment that self is on the throne of my heart and I am self-oriented. I do what I want to do because I want to do it. And let's say that I like driving my car fast, regardless of the speed limit. As long as I speed and get away with it, I see speeding as a gain.

But when I get caught, and I have to pay a fine, go to driving school, and pay a higher insurance premium—when I receive negative consequences to my decision—that consequence is a loss.

That one time of being caught and fined—of receiving negative consequences to my decision—may be enough for me to consider speeding a loss. But it may not. I may have to be caught several times and fined several times before I finally believe speeding to be a loss, but I only consider it to be a loss when I think I may be caught. I still enjoy speeding when I don't think anyone will catch me, so I drive with a radar detector, slow down when I see a police officer, etc. Or, I fear that I will be caught any time, and I drive under the speed limit for fear of ever being caught. But if I ever come to a place or time when I think I won't be caught, I speed, because it is still considered a gain.

But when I become God-oriented, when God is my greatest treasure, and when I learn the truth in Romans 13:1, "Let every soul be subject to the governing authorities. For there is no authority except from God, and the authorities that exist are appointed by

God," and when I understand that God is always aware of what I am doing, then I believe speeding is a loss, because it would be rebellion against God and the authorities that He has placed over me. It is not a temporary loss, dependent upon whether I will be caught or not. It is a permanent loss, because it is related to God, and God doesn't change.

Now, what if I were back at the beginning, living with a spouse who doesn't love me enough, and thinking that divorce is a lesser loss and infidelity is a gain compared to it. And there is some guy named Bob that I come into contact with. I don't know who Bob is, and he doesn't have any influence in my life. But Bob says that he hates adultery, and he hates divorce. Does that change my treasure so that I make decisions any differently? No, it doesn't. I could care less what Bob thinks. His thinking makes no impact upon my decisions, because he is not a treasure to me, and thus his opinion has no weight to change my treasure and thus my decisions. Bob doesn't have any influence in my heart, my treasure, or my decisions.

No one naturally likes to deny themselves. We all naturally like to indulge ourselves. It is a gain to us. So, since we always choose a gain over a loss, we will always choose indulgence over self-denial. But, if we learn (and believe) that to indulge self is to win a ticket to hell, then self-indulgence becomes a loss.

How much of a loss does it become? It becomes a loss in proportion to the loss that we consider hell to be. But what is the loss of hell? Hell represents the loss of eternal life, of heaven, of God's approval, the loss of an eternal relationship with God, angels, and friends, etc. So, the degree to which we treasure the things which we lose by gaining hell, is the degree to which hell is a loss to us.

Since the loss of hell is a greater loss than denying self, we will choose self-denial over self-indulgence in order to maintain our greater gains (eternal life, heaven, eternal relationship with God, God's approval, etc.) and avoid the loss of those treasures (hell). And by associating the loss of self-denial with the greater gain of God's favor, self-denial becomes a gain, and no longer a loss.

To do something that was perceived as a loss, you must: 1) adopt a greater loss as its alternative, or 2) believe it to be a gain by attaching it to a greater gain.

If, however, my greatest treasure is pleasure (sinful), then complete self-denial would be considered a loss. But lust would be considered a gain, for there is much pleasure associated with lust. And because lust was believed to be a gain (because it is associated with my treasure of pleasure), and complete self-denial was considered a loss, the heart would automatically choose lust over complete self-denial, because the heart always chooses a gain over a loss.

With pleasure (sinful) as my greatest treasure, I would believe complete self-denial to be a loss. And I would also consider partial self-denial as a loss. But to my sinful heart, partial self-denial is not as great of a loss as complete self-denial. So, in my sin-oriented heart, I could still choose partial self-denial, even though it is a loss to me. But I can only do so to avoid complete self-denial, which is a greater loss to me. So, with pleasure or sin as my treasure, I will choose lust or partial self-denial over complete self-denial.

But if pleasure and sin as a treasure are replaced by God and His favor, sin now becomes a loss, because it represents to me a loss of God's favor—my greatest treasure. To think, say, and do what is right becomes a gain to me, because it maintains my greatest treasure—God's favor. And so, by having God as my treasure, I will choose to think, say, and do that which is right, and I will avoid sin, because the heart always chooses a gain over a loss.

Now let us look at another aspect. No one likes to suffer. God never designed man to suffer, and suffering is the result of sin, but in the context of a sinful world, it is possible to suffer for God's sake—to standing for the right to gain or maintain the treasure of God. And if I believe suffering for God is a lesser loss than sin, I will choose suffering for God rather than sin, because we always choose a lesser loss over a greater one. But when I associate suffering for God with the retention of my greatest treasure—God's favor—then suffering becomes a gain. We see this in the life of Paul. "Yet indeed I also count all things loss for the excellence of the knowledge of Christ Jesus my Lord, for whom I have suffered the loss of all things, and count them as rubbish, that I may gain Christ."[58]

Previously in Paul's life, he considered many things to be gain (riches, man's approval, pleasure, self-righteousness, etc.). But when Christ became the greatest treasure of his life, those things which had been considered gain, but were actually contrary to Christ, were now considered loss, because they would cause the loss of his greatest treasure, which was Christ. Paul lost those things which at one time he had considered a gain, but now that Christ had become his greatest treasure, the loss of those things was no longer a loss, because he was losing losses (not treasures), and he was gaining his treasure (Christ).

So, with God as my greatest treasure, my will becomes aligned with God's will, and I automatically choose that which God would, because I treasure God. His valuation system becomes my valuation system, and I choose to think, say, and do what is right; I suffer for God, and I avoid sin, because He is my treasure.

With self as my greatest treasure, self-indulgence becomes my greatest gain. I do what I want to do, when I want to do it, and how I want it done for my own selfish reasons. Pride and selfishness are the underlying motivations of my life, and I see others as sources of what I need, so I orient myself to others in order to get that which I want or need. What others think and how they respond is important to me, because I believe I need what they have, and I find myself a slave

---

[58] Philippians 3:8

to others, trying to get what I need from them but never really being able to control them. Hurt, frustration, anger, manipulation, fighting, etc. are the result.

I can even put God into the same category, trying to manipulate Him to get from Him that which I think I want or need. But the motivation of my heart is still for self. I see God as a source of what I need, and so my selfishness seeks from Him the blessings. But I still do not value self-denial, and self is still the god on the throne of my heart. My service for God is not because He is on the throne, but because I see Him as a means to get what I want and need. My service to Him is a form of manipulation—a bartering tool, if you please—whereby I try to do the right things so that I can get the blessings. I see and treat God like a genie in a genie lamp, trying to rub the genie lamp just the right way so that I can get my wishes.

And if self is my greatest treasure, then self-denial, whether partial or complete, is not desirable. It is a loss. To be told that I can't eat the cake I want to indulge in, to not be allowed to take the car for a spin around the neighborhood with my friends when I want to, to let someone else get the promotion I have been waiting for, all of this is undesirable. All of this I avoid if possible. A self-oriented heart is the condition of sinful humanity.

But when God becomes the greatest treasure of my life, everything changes. Instead of being self-oriented, I become God-oriented. I am first and foremost concerned about what God wants, so I do what He wants, when He wants it, how He wants it, and I do it out of the motivation of love. The love of God is my motivation, and I see that self is in conflict with God, so I deny self to gain the greater treasure of God, and I see self-denial as a gain, because it is associated with the greater treasure.

I am no longer a slave to people, because I recognize that they are not my source, and they do not possess that which I need. God is my Source. He has all that I need. Others are there for me to give away that which I took from God. I am not oriented toward them in that I try to control or manipulate them to get what I need from them, but I am oriented toward them in that I enjoy helping them by giving to them that which I have taken from God. I love them because God loves them, and I love God. They are valuable to me because they are valuable to God. What they do with the gift is not my problem and doesn't personally affect me. I don't give to them to receive anything back. I do it because I have taken what I need from God and love to give it away. The result is love, joy, peace, patience, kindness, goodness, faithfulness, gentleness, and self-control—the fruit of the Spirit.

And my service for God is not a means to manipulate Him to get what I want or need. It is a grateful response to Him for the love and blessings He has already given to me. Love for God, not selfishness, becomes my motivation when God is my greatest treasure.

I want to highlight one last point here. When God is the greatest treasure of my life, anything that pertains to God, anything that is aligned with His will, anything that involves His kingdom is considered a gain. And anything that is against God, anything that is opposed to His will, anything that detracts from His kingdom is considered a loss. John puts it this way, "Do not love the world or the things in the world. If anyone loves the world, the love of the Father is not in him."[59] You cannot love the world (which is controlled by and in harmony with the Enemy) and the things of the world (the world's entertainment, fashions, possessions, pleasures, popularity, power, positions, and principles) when God is the greatest treasure of your heart—when God is your God. All of these things will be considered losses to the heart where God reigns.

But when sin and self is the greatest treasure of my life, anything that pertains to self and sin, anything that is aligned with the Enemy's

---

[59] 1 John 2:15

will, anything that involves the world and the things of the world is considered a gain. And anything that is against self and sin (righteousness, judgment, consequences, etc.), anything that is opposed to my will (humility, self-sacrifice, selfless love, etc.), and anything that denies me the world and the things of this world is considered a loss. You cannot love God and the things that pertain to His kingdom when self and sin is the greatest treasure of your heart—when self is your god. All of these things will be considered losses to the heart where self reigns. It is absolutely true that anyone who loves the world, "the love of the Father is not in him." And this is a problem of the heart—a problem of the treasure. And the only solution to it is a new heart.

"All true obedience comes from the heart. It was heart work with Christ. And if we consent, He will so identify Himself with our thoughts and aims, so blend our hearts and minds into conformity to His will, that when obeying Him we shall be but carrying out our own impulses. The will, refined and sanctified, will find its highest delight in doing His service. When we know God as it is our privilege to know Him, our life will be a life of continual obedience. Through an appreciation of the character of Christ, through communion with God, sin will become hateful to us."[60]

A change in one's beliefs leads to a change in one's valuation system, which leads to a change in one's choices, which leads to a change in one's behaviors or actions. But this change is only temporary. It is dependent upon what I believe, and what I believe can change. If I want a permanent change, I need another component.

A conviction leads to a change in one's valuation system, which leads to a change in one's choices, which leads to a change in one's behaviors or actions. And this change is permanent. It will not change regardless of threat or inducement. You can't get someone to change

[60] White, E.G. (1898) *The Desire of Ages.* (p 668). Review and Herald Publishing Association.

their mind from a conviction, for it is a permanent setting of the treasure in the heart, which results in a permanent setting of the decisions which are made based upon that treasure.

Revelation chapter 7 introduces us to the 144,000, who will be faithful to God in the end of time—those who are represented in Revelation 14:12 as "those who keep the commandments of God and the faith of Jesus." Revelation 7, verses 3 & 4 tell us that those who become the 144,000 are those who are sealed in their foreheads. What is this seal?

This seal is conviction based upon truth, so that we cannot be persuaded to change our minds or decisions regardless of the pressure we face. "Just as soon as the people of God are sealed in their foreheads,—it is not any seal or mark that can be seen, but a settling into the truth, both intellectually and spiritually, so they cannot be moved,—just as soon as God's people are sealed and prepared for the shaking, it will come. Indeed, it has begun already; the judgments of God are now upon the land, to give us warning, that we may know what is coming."[61]

That conviction, that seal, is so firm, that not even the threat of death will shake our decision or convince us to sin. "Those who would rather die than perform a wrong act are the only ones who will be found faithful."[62] This is the condition of the 144,000 who will be ready for the Lord's return, and this is a condition of the heart, of the treasure, based upon conviction. This is the condition that I want to be settling into now, don't you?

So, being convicted that God is the greatest treasure of my life permanently aligns my will with the will of God, and I will not sin, because I permanently see sin as the greatest loss (although it still offers pleasure, power, position, prestige, etc.) because it represents

---

[61] White, E.G. (1981) *Manuscript Releases Volume One.* (p 249). Silver Spring, MD: Ellen G. White Estate.
[62] White, E.G. (1889) *Testimonies for the Church, Volume 5.* (p 53). Mountain View, CA: Pacific Press Publishing Association.

the loss of my greatest treasure. That conviction is so strong, that even the threat of death will not move me to sin. I am settled into the truth. God is my treasure. And nothing can change that.

So, how do I make God my treasure? First of all, I can read God's word with the purpose to know Him and to love Him. Don't read just for the accumulation of information. Read for the purpose of understanding who God is, what He is like, how His character is revealed, and what a relationship with Him is like.

Secondly, I can spend frequent, earnest time in prayer. Just like any relationship, it takes time. Make it your habit to begin the day with prayer before any other thoughts or distractions occupy your mind. Go out in nature and earnestly, passionately, seek to know Him. Speak to Him of your difficulties and troubles. Ask Him to answer your prayers. Keep a journal of your discussions with God, requests made of Him, and answers to those requests. Give Him thanks for the blessings in your life. Simply speak to Him as you would speak with a friend.

Thirdly, contemplate the life of Christ, especially the closing scenes of His life. Think about what it was like to be with Him in each of the stories you read. Think about what each of the characters in the story might have been thinking or feeling. Think about the love that Jesus was manifesting at the time. And especially try to understand how much love went into His sacrifice from the garden of Gethsemane to the cross. There, you will see most clearly the amazing love of God. And seeing and knowing that love with create within you a love for God.

Fourth, contemplate the blessings of God. Contemplate what it means to be forgiven of all of your sins and made perfect before God because of His sacrifice for you. Contemplate what heaven will be like and the eternal joys and discoveries of the universe. Contemplate what it will be like to be with Jesus throughout all eternity, growing in relationship with Him and others. Contemplate what a blessing His sacrificial life has been and will continue to be in your life.

Fifth, recount, test, and believe His promises. Search the Bible for promises that address the issues you are facing and read them frequently, write them down, memorize them, test them out in different circumstances, and bend every effort of your mind to believe them.

And sixth, ask the Holy Spirit to make God your treasure, and then cooperate with His working in your heart, allowing Him full access to accomplish it in you.

"Again, the kingdom of heaven is like treasure hidden in a field, which a man found and hid; and for joy over it he goes and sells all that he has and buys that field."[63] "Again, the kingdom of heaven is like a merchant seeking beautiful pearls, who, when he had found one pearl of great price, went and sold all that he had and bought it."[64] "It is the Holy Spirit that reveals to men the preciousness of the goodly pearl. The time of the Holy Spirit's power is the time when in a special sense the heavenly gift is sought and found."[65]

A Treasured Experience

For those who are seeking for the hidden treasure and the Pearl of great price (Matthew 13:44-46), I want to encourage you with my testimony.

I have sought this treasure my whole life, sometimes with greater passion and sometimes with less. I sought it through church. I sought it through prayer. I sought it through Bible study. I sought it through acts of service. I sought it in many places and at varied times throughout my life, but until recently, I have not seen the treasure for what it really is.

---

[63] Matthew 13:44
[64] Matthew 13:45,46
[65] White, E. G. (1900) *Christ's Object Lessons.* (p. 118). Review and Herald Publishing Association.

The Lord has been so good to me throughout the years. He has revealed Himself to me in prayer. He has revealed Himself to me in His word. And He has revealed Himself to me through others. He has pursued me all of my life (Luke 15). He is an awesome God who loves me so much (John 3:16). But for most of my life, I was not willing to surrender to Him completely. I always reserved something for myself.

About 10 years ago, the Lord allowed me to come to a very dark and desperate time in my life—a time when I finally gave up. I was destroying myself and the ones that I loved, and I could see that I had no power to break free from that which held me in bondage (Romans 7:15-24). In my desperation God asked me to turn my entire life over to Him, to let Him be in control (Matthew 11:28-30, Luke 9:23). That was a scary prospect to me, because I had always been in control. I didn't know if I could trust God or not. But finally, with no hope in myself, with no ability to get myself out of the mess I was in, I decided to give everything over to Him.

"Lord, I will do anything that you ask me to do, no matter how embarrassing or painful. I will go wherever you want me to go, no matter how reluctant I feel. I will give up whatever you ask for, no matter how precious it seems to me. If following you means I lose my family, I will follow. If it means being embarrassed, I will follow. If it means the loss of my career, reputation, or even the loss of my abilities, I will follow. Whatever you ask for, I will do it. Just get me out of this mess."

God presented to me a picture of a tightrope drawn across a canyon, and Jesus, as the expert tightrope artist, was standing there with a wheelbarrow balanced on the line, the handles firmly held in His hands. And He called me to get into the wheelbarrow (Matthew 19:21). On my own, all I could do was fall over the edge of the canyon to certain death below (Romans 3:23; 6:23). But in His wheelbarrow (which to my mind represented faith and complete surrender), there was a chance that He could get me safely across the canyon (John 6:39).

As He called to me to get into the wheelbarrow, I struggled, seeing that at any time that I started to take over control again, the wheelbarrow would tip, and I would fall out (Matthew 14:30). I saw that once I got in, I would either stay in or fall to my death. I saw that I would have to give up control of my life for good (Romans 6:16). And I wasn't sure if I could trust Jesus with that kind of control. He reminded me that I would certainly destroy myself if I remained in control of my life (Jeremiah 17:9), and He again, gently invited me into His wheelbarrow. I finally got into the wheelbarrow, and life has never been the same!

I found that He has a thousand ways to free me from that which I couldn't find a single way of escape from (Hebrews 7:25). I found that all the things I had forced myself to do before to come to Jesus (prayer, Bible study, service, obedience) were the very things that I now did naturally, willingly, and with joy (Romans 8:26,27). Life was new, different, exciting, liberating, and victorious.

As time progressed, I became more and more consistent with prayer and study of His word. My habits and preferences changed. My diet, entertainment, dress, recreation, friends, desires, and thoughts changed. God was making me into a new creation in Christ Jesus (2 Corinthians 5:17).

Over the last few years, the Lord has brought me to a place of consistency in prayer. Regardless of how I feel or how much I want to just "become one" with my bed, I get up in the early mornings to spend time with the Lord in prayer. He has been revealing much to me regarding His love over the last several years, and the ideas of His love and mercy have grown in my mind (Ephesians 3:17-19). I have had the privilege to teach thousands of people about this love, and each time I teach it, I learn more and more about it.

Each Wednesday I pray and fast with a few individuals, where we take our lunch period and spend it together praying, rather than eating. It has been an encouragement to me to be involved in this with others, seeking our Lord together and bringing our petitions and challenges before Him (Matthew 18:19,20). The episode that I will mention next happened on a Thursday morning after the Wednesday prayer and fast. I believe there is a connection.

One Thursday morning, as is my custom, I woke up early, got dressed, and went outside to walk and pray (I find that I can't fall asleep while I am walking, and when I am very tired it is very easy for me to fall asleep during prayer). As I walked out of the house and looked up into the sky, I saw thousands of stars shining down upon me.

The day before had not been a very good day, and the first thing on my agenda for prayer time that morning, after praising God for life and another day with the opportunities that it provided (Psalm 9:1), was to ask for forgiveness for my attitude and responses the previous day (1 John 1:9). Yet again, I had misrepresented the Lord and taken things into my own hands. During the couple weeks before this time, I had been convicted that I needed to get back into the wheelbarrow (Proverbs 24:16), and the Lord was showing me more clearly how to get back in. For about a week, also, I felt convicted that I didn't have any belief of my own and that I needed God to give me belief so that I could believe (Mark 9:24). Also, I had been studying about the hidden treasure and the pearl of great price, and I started thinking about that treasure—that pearl—which is Jesus (Matthew 13:44-46).

As I was outside in the dark of the morning with the stars shining down upon me, I prayed earnestly to the Lord to give me the gift of belief so that I could believe that Jesus was really worth to me as much as He is worth.

Under those stars, I began to think about how large they were and how much distance was between them. I thought about how long it would take to travel to the nearest star and then across our Milky Way Galaxy. I thought about how vast was the universe that we can see, realizing that there is infinity beyond what we can see. I thought about the fact that God is larger, not smaller, than His creation, and that a God infinitely big is also a God that is infinitely powerful (Psalm 89:8). I thought about that God loving such a small and insignificant creature like me.

I thought about that infinite God loving me so much that He chose to come to this infinitesimally small planet to rescue me. I thought about that infinite God packaging Himself inside a single cell in Mary's womb, becoming the smallest and most vulnerable form of life. And for what? For me (John 3:16)!

The Holy Spirit was working upon my heart, giving me the gift of belief as I continued to think about how precious Jesus is. I thought about the fact that it is the character of God to give (Matthew 5:45); and that His joy is found in giving. And yet, when it came to the ransom of a rebel world, it took three meetings between Jesus and the Father before the Father consented to give His Son as the ransom for our race. If God's nature is to give, but He wavered at giving the gift of Jesus, then how great is that gift?!

With a realizing sense of the greatness of that gift given on my behalf, with a realizing sense of how precious Jesus is and how infinitely valuable He is, I was overwhelmed by the thought and just began to weep and fell to my knees in the dirt. All I could think of and pray/cry at the time was, "Who am I that You would give such a Gift for me? Who am I that you would give Jesus for me? Who am I?"

Lost in the wonder of that overwhelming thought, the only appropriate response that I could think of was, "Thank You! Thank You! Thank You!" After a couple minutes, I picked myself off the ground, dusted off my clothes, and continued to walk and just revel in the thought of the infinite love of God for me. As I walked in the dark of the early morning, it was as if I was walking just outside of the gates of Heaven. It was a most singular and wonderful experience. I had never experienced anything like that before.

I began to think about Moses and his experience with God. He desired to see God, so God put him in the cleft of the rock, held His hand over him, and passed by him with His back toward Moses (Exodus 33:18-23; 34:5-8). He revealed to Moses all of the glory that Moses could handle. I felt that the Lord was revealing His glory to me to the degree that I could handle. It was beautiful, just beautiful!

I knew that this was a gift from God, that He had given me the gift of belief so that I could believe that Jesus was as precious as He really was. And when I believed, everything changed. I walked over to my car, and laid down on the trunk, staring up at the stars in the sky and thinking about how great and wonderful God is and how infinite His love is to me. Again, I began to cry at the thought that such a love existed, and that it was exercised for me.

I thought of the sacrifice of Jesus. I thought of how He was misunderstood, taken advantage of, rejected, scorned, derided, beaten, nailed to a cross, separated from His father, and apparently forsaken—all for me! I thought of how much He loved those whom He came to save (Romans 5:8), and how many walked away from the eternal gift He came to give (John 6:66). I thought of how much it must have hurt the heart of God for His infinite love to be rejected like that. I thought of how much Jesus loved each of the ones He came to save, and how much it must have tortured His heart when His children rejected His Father's love (not that He hurt for Himself, because He didn't, but that He hurt for them and what that rejection meant to them).

Then I thought about all of the times that I had rejected His love for me and chose to do my own thing. I began to cry again at the thought of the pain I had caused the Lord through my willful disobedience and love of sin. How hateful sin became to me in that

moment! It defied the God who loved me so much. It separated me
from Him so that He couldn't accomplish in my life that which He
desired to accomplish. It harmed and killed the children He loved so
much that He left all of heaven to rescue them. How could I possibly
love sin in the face of such love—in the face of the infinite
preciousness of Jesus?

I got up from the car and began to walk again, and as I walked, I
thought about what sin had to offer. Sin offered power, positions,
possessions, pleasure, and popularity. But next to Jesus, none of
those things mattered at all. It was as if each of those things were
worth between $1,000 and $10,000, and depending upon my
personality and desires, the value of each of those things varied
accordingly. I might desire pleasure over popularity, position over
possessions, etc. And to me, pleasure might be sin's greatest gain,
which was symbolically worth $10,000. But Jesus was worth
$1,000,000,000,000,000,000,000 in comparison. I had always known
this intellectually, but now that God gave me the gift of belief, I
actually believed it.

I realized that sin had nothing to offer me, and in that moment—
believing that Jesus was worth how much He is worth—sin had no
attraction to me. Thinking about anything that had been a temptation
to me before, none of it had any appeal or attraction to me now. I
saw that in the full realization of who Jesus is and how precious He is,
sin loses its power to attract and tempt (Philippians 3:7,8). In that
moment, sin had no power over me, no attraction to me, was no
temptation to me. (Psalm 17:3) Why? Because the infinite value of
Jesus was presented to me in unmistakable clarity and I believed it.
And in the realization of that infinite value of Jesus, I died to sin
(Romans 6:10), for it only offered to me a loss of Jesus, which was a
loss of all things (Philippians 3:8).

Thinking of how infinitely precious Jesus was, my heart was
changed. I no longer desired sin. I no longer found difficulty in

obeying God. I delighted in His law and following His will (Psalm 40:8). I had no attraction to sin and this world, but was intensely attracted to Jesus and heaven (Romans 6:16. "When the sinner has a view of the matchless charms of Jesus, sin no longer looks attractive to him; for he beholds the Chiefest among ten thousand, the One altogether lovely. He realizes by a personal experience the power of the gospel, whose vastness of design is equaled only by its preciousness of purpose."[66]).

Again, it felt as if I was walking just outside the gates of heaven, and I couldn't help but think again, "Lord, who am I that you would reveal such beautiful truth to me? Who am I that you would give me such an experience? Who am I?" Several times I just stopped walking, caught up in the wonder of the thought of the infinite worth of Christ and what it meant in relation to everything else in life.

I then began to think about the bad things in life. What if I lost LeEtta (my wife)? What if I lost my children (I have six)? What if there was a fire and the house burned and we lost all we had? What if I lost my job and could never work in my career again (I am a missionary physician)? What if I was injured or sick and was paralyzed and could do nothing, needing others to take care of me? What if I was taken captive and tortured because of my faith? All of these scenarios ran through my mind, but to each scenario, my response was the same—it wouldn't matter. It simply wouldn't matter. I would still have Jesus, and He was infinitely valuable.

The loss of anything and everything that I had was nothing in comparison to having Jesus. If I lost it all, but still had Jesus, I would be completely okay. In contemplating each of these potential challenges, I had perfect peace and a joy that was beyond description (Romans 15:13). I realized that I could face the loss of all things and undergo physical torture and still have perfect peace and abundant joy. I didn't just know it intellectually; I truly experienced it that

---

[66] White, E. G. (1892) Accepted in Christ. *The Signs of the Times.* July 4, 1892, paragraph 5.

morning. God gave me a glimpse into what could be by giving me the gift of belief to believe that Jesus was all to me that He actually is.

In that state of mind—in the midst of that experience—I again realized that sin had absolutely no attraction to me and that there was nothing, absolutely nothing, that could disturb the peace that I felt at the time, because Jesus was my infinite treasure. I realized that this was the experience of Jesus as He lived in human flesh. He was never attracted to sin. It was always repulsive to Him, because it meant the loss of all things—the loss of His Father. Nothing could disturb His peace, because nothing could separate Him from His father (until He became sin for us before the cross – 2 Corinthians 5:21). So, His life was one of peace, joy, and complete victory over sin.

And for a few moments, God permitted me to enter into that experience too. It was a gift—a gift of God's grace to a sinful child of His who has been seeking to know and love God. As the moments rolled on, I could feel the experience fading. I just kept telling God, "I love this experience. Thank you so much for revealing this to me. I want more! I want this to not be the only experience of this nature and magnitude."

Moses had that initial experience with God in the mountain, but his walk with God grew and he was permitted to talk face to face with God. God came so close to him that Moses's own face glowed with a radiance that was painful to those who looked upon him (Exodus 34:29-35). I pleaded that the Lord would continue to reveal Himself to me more and more consistently and more and more profoundly, so that I could remain in this experience consistently.

"I want more and more of you, Jesus. I want to know that you are as precious as you are. I ask for a heart to believe that You are worth what You are worth. I want to be held by you in peace, joy, and complete victory over sin, because You are the infinite treasure of my heart. Keep me by your love in your love, that I might abide in You, the Vine (John 15:4)."

CHAPTER SIX

Leaving Your Baggage Behind

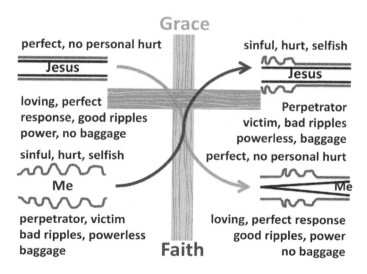

Double Crossed

Y ou and I have a past, and each past is unique. None of us have been through the exact same difficulties and trials, and yet there are many similarities in our experiences. Unfortunately, that past has the tendency to determine the direction of our life in the future. Why unfortunately? It is because most of our past experiences direct us in the wrong path—send us in the wrong direction.

What do we do about the past? Is there a solution to the things we have already suffered? Is there freedom from the baggage that we have carried with us for years and years? There is. And the solution is found at the cross.

Jesus, the unwearied servant of man's necessity, the One who poured himself into hurting humanity to raise us up from the fall, the One who sacrificed all heaven and the constant adoration of the angelic host, the One who created all creatures great and small, the One who came to reveal God to man and restore the breach made by sin; Jesus bore our sin. No, more than this, He *became* our sin. And He did so that we might become His righteousness.

"The spotless Son of God hung upon the cross, His flesh lacerated with stripes; those hands so often reached out in blessing, nailed to the wooden bars; those feet so tireless on ministries of love, spiked to the tree; that royal head pierced by the crown of thorns; those quivering lips shaped to the cry of woe. And all that He endured—the blood drops that flowed from His head, His hands, His feet, the agony that racked His frame, and the unutterable anguish that filled His soul at the hiding of His Father's face—speaks to each child of humanity, declaring, It is for thee that the Son of God consents to bear this burden of guilt; for thee He spoils the domain of death, and opens the gates of Paradise. He who stilled the angry waves and walked the foam-capped billows, who made devils tremble and disease flee, who opened blind eyes and called forth the dead to life,—offers Himself upon the cross as a sacrifice, and this from love to thee. He, the Sin Bearer, endures the wrath of divine justice, and for thy sake becomes sin itself."[67]

[67] White, E. G. (1898) *The Desire of Ages*. (p 755). Review and Herald Publishing Association.

It is one thing to carry sin. I can faintly understand the concept of bearing or carrying sin. But to become sin? This I can't comprehend. To think that Jesus, the Son of God, who had never been separated from His father in the span of all eternity, became in some way became the very thing that His Father hated—the very thing that separates us from God. But why? Why would He do it? He did it because He wanted to accomplish something equally incomprehensible.

He tells us in 2 Corinthians 5:21, "For He made Him who knew no sin to be sin for us, that we might become the righteousness of God in Him." Here we are told the reason He became sin. He did so that we might *become* the righteousness of God *in Him*. I can't comprehend this either. I know myself. I know how much I fail. I know my wandering thoughts, mistakes, and rebellions. I know my stubborn will. And yet Jesus became sin so that I could *become* the righteousness of God! I do not mean to say that Jesus was ever guilty of sin or ever committed sin, but that in some "alien" way, He was permitted to become sin, so that I, in a similar "alien" way might become the righteousness of God *in Him*. What amazing love He has for me! But, in order to accomplish this incomprehensible feat, He had to go to the cross.

Before the Cross

What was the life of Christ like before the cross? Was He fully God? Yes. Was He fully man? Yes. He had a dual nature. And He was perfect. How full of perfection is perfect? Completely full. So, how much room was there for sin in His life? There was no room for even a single sin.

He had no personal hurts. He was like the UPS delivery guy, bringing His Father's love to those He came into contact with. And if that love was rejected, He didn't take it personally—even once! Yes, He hurt, but He hurt for others, not Himself. He was loving with an unselfish, self-sacrificing love. He always responded perfectly to anything that happened to Him even though many things happened to Him that were bad. He had power from His Father to overcome all temptation and sin. And he had good ripples.

What do I mean by good ripples? If you throw a pebble into a pond, the initial splash of the pebble swells into ever-increasing ripples that travel much farther than the original impact. Ripples represent not just what was said and done, but the influence that those things had upon others. Because of who Jesus was and how He lived, every word and action of His life resulted in ripples that travel through all time and space and positively impact every creature that has ever lived. Adam and Eve benefitted by His ripples, and you and I benefit from them today. Even the angels benefit from the ripples of the life of Christ. Because of His perfect life and the perfect influence that it had, Jesus had no baggage. And that life earns the blessing of eternal life.

But what about you and me? What is our life like before the cross? We look a little bit different from Him. In fact, to find a correct description of our character, what we need to do is take any true description of Christ and go to a thesaurus and find the section called "antonyms." There we will find a correct description of ourselves. Christ was perfect, with no room for sin. We are sinful, with no room for righteousness.

Christ was *never* personally hurt by what others said or did. We *always* take what others say and do personally. Christ had a selfless, self-sacrificing love. We have a selfish "love," which is why we take things personally and take things into our own hands.

Christ always responded perfectly to every person and situation. We have acted poorly toward others, hurting them by our words, actions, or influence. And we are victims, having had many things happen to us that we had no control over, and which we responded poorly to. Christ had power to overcome every temptation and sin.

We are powerless to truly overcome any temptation and sin from a pure motive, therefore our "overcoming" temptation is through bad motives, which itself is sin.

Instead of having good ripples, we have bad ripples. If you ever wonder about whether you have bad ripples, just have children. In them you will see the sure effects of your influence as your tendencies and weaknesses are manifested in them. The things we say and do have a negative impact or influence upon others beyond our children also. And you can never get those bad ripples back. Every time you try to catch the bad ripples, you make new ones that spread even farther. And all this fills our heavy suitcase, which is our baggage. And this life earns the penalty of death.

Humanity is so enslaved by our past. It is as if our past experience drives our future trajectory. It is like the experiences of the past form the gun barrel of our lives, and the bullet of our lives always travels in the direction of that gun barrel. Those who were abused as a child have a tendency to become abusers when they grow up.

The Sanctuary Service

So, what did Jesus offer us at the cross? What did He accomplish there? To understand this, we first need to understand the cross in the larger context of the plan of redemption as outlined in the sanctuary service of the Old Testament.

What was the purpose of the sanctuary service of the Old Testament? One purpose was to reveal to us how God intended to take care of the sin problem.

If an individual sinned, he would bring an unblemished sacrifice (lamb, goat, bull, etc.—see Leviticus Chapter 4) to the sanctuary in the center of the Israelite camp. Once inside the outer court, he would lay his hand upon the head of the animal and confess his sin(s) over it and then slit its throat with a knife.

The blood from the lamb would be caught in a bowl by the priest and carried to the alter of burnt offering in the outer court and put on the four horns of the altar. A similar sacrifice would be made by the priest in the morning and evening for the sins of Israel, and this time the blood was taken by the priest to the holy place of the sanctuary and placed on the four horns of the altar of incense. In figure, the sin was transferred from the sinner, to the sacrificial animal, to the priest, and then to the sanctuary.

Once a year, a ceremony was performed on the Day of Atonement (see Leviticus chapter 16), where two goats were brought to the outer court and a lot was cast to see which one would be the Lord's goat and which one would be the scapegoat. The Lord's goat and a bull were killed in similar fashion, and this time, the high priest would take the blood all the way into the most holy place of the sanctuary.

The ark of the covenant, which was the only furniture in the most holy place, was a gold-covered box that contained the ten commandments—the law of God. On top of this box were two intricately carved angels, and between the angels on the center of the box was a golden lid, or seat, called the mercy seat. This is where the presence of God resided in the temple.

The high priest would come into the most holy place once a year, on the Day of Atonement, and sprinkle the blood on the mercy seat. He would then walk out to the outer court, lay his hands on the head of the scapegoat, confess the sins of Israel that had accumulated in the sanctuary for the entire year, and then have the scapegoat led out into the desert to die alone and never return to the camp of Israel.

This illustrates how God is going to take care of the sin problem. The sinner confesses his sin, Jesus (the Lamb of God) takes that sin as His own (from the end of the last supper until His death on the cross) and dies under its penalty. Jesus, after He resurrected to new life and returned to heaven, is now our High Priest, officiating in the heavenly sanctuary (see the book of Hebrews). As our High Priest, He takes our confessed sins, which His own blood paid for 2,000 years ago, and transfers them to the heavenly sanctuary, awaiting the day when the accumulated sins will be placed upon Satan—the instigator of sin—and Satan will pay for all the sin he caused God's children commit. And when Satan is destroyed, sin will be destroyed with him. This is God's plan to take care of sin.

At/After the Cross

So, on the cross, Jesus takes our place. He steps into the gun barrel of our lives and takes the bullet that our lives have deserved. He takes the responsibility for our sinfulness and selfishness. He takes the results of us taking things personally. He takes the penalty of being the perpetrator and the consequences of being the victim. He takes the powerlessness of human flesh to overcome temptation and sin. He not only takes the responsibility for the things that were said and done, but He also takes the responsibility for the ripples—the negative influence and effects that those things have had and will have on others. He takes our baggage for us. The death that our life deserves, Jesus suffers.

In addition to doing all of this, Jesus does something else. As Jesus steps into the gun barrel of our lives and takes the force of all that it deserves, He gently places us in the gun barrel of His life. When He does so, we receive eternal life and all of the other blessings and benefits that His perfect life deserved. And the gun barrel of His life guides the bullet directly to the bulls-eye of the target, which is holiness. We receive His power to overcome all temptation and sin. We no longer have to be controlled by our past and our negative responses. We can be controlled by Jesus past and His perfect responses, filled with His power.

When we enter into the experience of this divine exchange of life for life, history for history, past for past—offered to us because of God's sacrifice at the cross—Jesus' record becomes ours in the books of heaven. We are accounted perfect. We have no personal hurts. We are perfectly loving. We have responded perfectly to everything that has happened to us in the past. We have power to overcome. We have perfect ripples that have spread through all time and space and have positively influenced everyone that those ripples have come into contact with. And we no longer have any baggage.

Jesus tells us, "Assuredly, I say to you, inasmuch as you did it to one of the least of these My brethren, you did it to Me."[68] This means that if you do it to someone else, you did it to Him. But it is equally true that if they did it to you, they did it to Jesus. Jesus so identifies Himself with us and our hurts and sins, that He, in a very real way, takes our place. It is as if those things which were done to us were actually done to Him.

On the cross, God offers us a divine exchange of life for life. This divine exchange is only made possible by God's grace. The price He paid on the cross was the price for each of our sins. He suffered under not only the weight of the world, but of each and every specific sin that you and I have ever committed or will ever commit. He paid the price for everyone who would accept the gift, and He paid the price for everyone who would reject the gift. He paid the price for us all.

But just because He paid the price for everyone doesn't mean that all will benefit from that gift. There will be many who are lost, for as yet, there is a part of the equation missing.

Faith is necessary in order for the gift of Grace to become mine. You see, the gift of this divine exchange of life for life is just like the buffet of God's love. He has made it free and available to each of us, but if we don't personally take of what has been provided, it does us

---

[68] Matthew 25:40

no good. Faith is our action that takes of what God provided and makes it our own. It is believing that God's gift of this divine exchange is for me. It is accepting that gift as my own and trusting that it is true for me, now. "For God so loved the world that He gave His only begotten Son, that whoever *believes* in Him should not perish but have everlasting life."[69]

What does this exchange look like in real life? Let us imagine that years ago you were in an argument with someone and the argument became so heated that the next thing you realize, the other person is lying dead on the floor. You killed them! You think, "Uh, oh! This isn't good. I don't want to go to prison." So, you get rid of the evidence, and you get away with it. No one discovers that you were the murderer. You are free, right? Wrong. You may be free in body, but you are a slave in your mind, always afraid if someone will find out, always encompassed by guilt.

But let us imagine that today you find out about this divine exchange made possible for you at the cross. You realize that Jesus is offering to step into the timeline of your life and take the consequences of the murder and all of the guilt and fear that came because of it and pay the penalty that you deserve. In exchange, you get placed into the timeline of His life, and you get all the consequences of His perfect life and the perfect ripples that it has created throughout all time and space.

You decide that you want to receive this gift, and faith accepts that gift made possible by grace. You accept it as your very own, believing that you are the recipient of all that Jesus' life deserved, while He took all the penalty of all that your life deserved. Your sin is then transferred by the Heavenly Priest, Jesus, to the heavenly sanctuary, awaiting the day when it will be placed upon the scapegoat, Satan, and be destroyed with him. You also confess your sin to those

---

[69] John 3:16

who were injured by it (family of the one murdered, etc.), and "come clean" on what you did.

After you enter into this divine exchange, where does the guilt of the murder lie? Not with you. It is in the heavenly sanctuary, awaiting the day when it will be placed upon Satan for him to pay for. You go free from the guilt.

If the family seeks for justice and reports the murder to the police before you get a chance to do so, and the investigation finds you "guilty," and you are placed in prison, according to heaven's record, are you guilty? No! You are innocent, because the guilt has been taken from you by the sacrifice made in your behalf on the cross. When you are placed in prison for the crime, you can be totally free in your mind, knowing that you are innocent in heaven's record.

You find yourself in the exact opposite situation than before coming to the cross. Before, you were free in the body and captive in the mind. Now you are free in the mind, but captive in the body. And that is a much better freedom. Like Paul and Silas, you can sing praises and hymns to Jesus in your imprisonment with a consciousness of your innocence because of the gift given to you at the cross.

Not only does the cross free us from what we did to others, it also frees us from what others did to us. There is not one of us who has had perfect parents. We have not had perfect family members. We have not had perfect friends. And because of this, we find ourselves the unwilling victims of what others have said and done.

In my position, I have the opportunity to hear many stories from people. Sometimes I am the only one that they have ever shared their secret with. Others have kept their story within the confines of a small circle of confidants. I have heard stories of abandonment, abuse, neglect, torture, rejection, divorce, and much more, and I know that I have only heard a small part of the pain that is out there.

I know that in a group as small as 5 people, there is likely to be one in the group who was sexually abused as a child. I know that within a group of as small as 2 married couples, one marriage will end in divorce. And I know that within a group as small as 1, there *is* a history of rejection, hurt, disappointment, etc. It is our universal experience in this world of sin.

So, let us imagine that you have been neglected, abused, rejected, abandoned, and mistreated in the past. Let us imagine that it is hard for you to get along with—much less love—the one(s) who did it to you. Let us imagine that you have carried, to one extent or another, resentment, hurt, shame, and/or bitterness, and as many times as you have tried to let it go, when you look again, it is still there.

And then today, you find out about the cross. You find out that God made it possible for you to go free from all of it. Jesus offers to step into the timeline of your life—your gun barrel—and take the brunt of the resentment, hurt, shame, bitterness, and all that was done to you and the death that it deserves. And in doing so, He gently nudges you into the timeline of His life—His gun barrel—and you get all of the blessings that His life deserved, including a clear record and eternal life. In contemplating this unfair exchange, you wonder, "How could it be?" and Jesus answers, "Assuredly, I say to you, inasmuch as you did it to one of the least of these My brethren, you did it to Me."[70]

You realize that if you do it to someone else, it is done to Jesus, so it must also be true that if someone else does it to you, they do it to Jesus, and therefore if it is done to you, it is done to Jesus. So, Jesus takes your place, and in doing so, He who was able to say, "Father, forgive them, for they do not know what they do,"[71] is also able to forgive those who treated Him so badly (when they treated Him badly through you).

---

[70] Matthew 25:40
[71] Luke 23:34

When I believe myself to be the victim of what others have said and done, I have lots of baggage. There is a lot that weighs me down. I may have attempted to forgive, but the roots of bitterness are still alive deep in my heart. When I think about them and what they did, I have hurt feelings and painful memories. The only way that I seem to get away from it is to try not to think about it. If I succeed in not thinking about it, I'll be okay, right? Wrong! Freedom doesn't come from a vacuum, and to simply not think about something is an attempt to create a vacuum.

Now imagine that you are doing prison ministries. You go to the prison and mix with the prisoners and minister to them. The people you work with are rapists, addicts, thieves, and murderers, but you can work with them just fine and love them. Why? Because they didn't do it to you. They didn't do it to your loved one. In prison ministries, you can relatively easily love those who hurt others, because they didn't do it to you.

There is a family that I know of, whose 11-year-old daughter went missing one day. It was in the days before cell phones, and parents kept track of their children by time. If you didn't come home by a certain time, you were in trouble, because your parents wanted to know that you were safe.

Well, she didn't come home on time, so her mother called the school. The school said that she left after school and headed toward home. Mother then called friends, and they confirmed that they saw her leaving school, walking toward home. Next Mother called Father, and he left work early to look for her.

He drove the street while Mother stayed at home awaiting her arrival. But she never came. As the shadows began to stretch across the fields, and as the sun fell below the tree line and darkness began to spread across the land, their hearts sank as they made the phone call they never thought they would make. They called 9-1-1 and told the operator, "We have a missing child."

First one officer was dispatched, and then others, and by the morning, as the search team grew, so did their hopes. But as the sun set each evening, their hopes of finding her died a little more, and each morning as they continued the search, their hopes rose less than the day before. A couple weeks later they received the word...one of the search teams had found her remains in the woods. The nightmare that they never dreamed they would have became the nightmare they would never wake up from. Hope died its last death. Their daughter would never come home.

As the investigation continued, the horror of the situation unfolded. It was revealed that a neighbor with a criminal record had abducted their daughter, treated her like bad people treat young girls, and then did the unspeakable, hiding her remains in the woods where the search dogs eventually found her. You can only imagine what was going on in the heart of that mother and father.

Now, let's imagine that that family had been accustomed to doing prison ministries, and one day they are at the prison, and they meet him there. How easy will it be for them to love him and minister to him? I tell you; it would be impossible. Why? Because what he did, he did to them and theirs.

The same is true of you and me. Others have done bad things to us and ours, and it is impossible for us to love them because we are the victim. At the cross, Jesus provided a way that we could escape from our past. He steps into the timeline of our lives and takes all that it entails, and He nudges us off into the timeline of His life and gives us all that it deserved. We don't have to be personally hurt by what was done, because after entering into the experience of the cross, Jesus takes our place. And just like prison ministries, we can love them and work for them and serve them, because they did it to Jesus, and He loves them and He offers them forgiveness.

Because I have entered into this experience of the cross, I love Jesus. And because Jesus loves them, I love them too. And if He is willing to sacrifice Himself for them, I am willing to do the same, because I have taken (accepted) that love and forgiveness for myself and am now just giving it away.

You see, God has a plan to save us from the current emotional hurts that we suffer. That plan involves giving us a new heart—by grace through faith. God also has a plan to save us from our past baggage. That plan involves the divine exchange made possible at the cross—by grace through faith.

Now, I want to point out one more truth that the cross teaches us. Before the cross, who is the unwilling victim who responds negatively to what was done? I am. After the cross, am I still the unwilling victim who responds negatively to what was done? No! That history and guilt and responsibility is transferred by Jesus our heavenly high priest, through the blood Jesus shed upon the cross, to the heavenly sanctuary awaiting the day when it will be placed upon Satan, who will pay for all of what he instigated.

In entering the experience of the cross, I can no longer remain the unwilling victim. And all of the negative feelings and thoughts associated with that victimhood (resentment, bitterness, anger, shame, etc.) can no longer stay with me. It is taken away from me by Jesus. I go free!

Now, I want to make this following point clear. If you are still the victim, you are living in an experience before the cross. You cannot come to the cross and remain the victim. Jesus, at the cross, sets you free from your past. But if you are not free from your past—if you are still the victim—it is because you have not come to the cross and accepted by faith the divine exchange made possible for you by God's grace. You are still bearing your burdens. You are still bearing your guilt. You cannot come to the cross and accept the divine exchange on your behalf and still be the victim.

Before the cross, who is the perpetrator? I am. After the cross, am I still guilty of being the perpetrator? No! That guilt and responsibility is transferred by Jesus our heavenly high priest, through the blood Jesus shed upon the cross, to the heavenly sanctuary awaiting the day when it will be placed upon Satan, who will pay for all that he instigated. In entering the experience of the cross, I can no longer remain guilty of the perpetrator's acts. And all of the negative feelings and thoughts associated with being the perpetrator (guilt, remorse, self-hatred, etc.) can no longer stay with me, because it is taken away from me by Jesus. I go free!

Now, if you are still holding on to the guilt of the perpetrator, you are living in an experience before the cross. You cannot come to the cross and retain the guilt of the perpetrator. Jesus, at the cross, sets you free from your past. But if you are not free from your past—if you are still the perpetrator—it is because you have not come to the cross, as it is your privilege, and accepted by faith the divine exchange made possible for you by God's grace. You are still bearing your burdens. You are still bearing your guilt. You cannot come to the cross and accept the divine exchange on your behalf and still be the perpetrator.

Forgiven?

How much of your sin did Jesus pay for on the cross? All of it! Did that include everything that you have ever done? Yes! Does that include everything that you will ever do? Yes!

How much of your life is God aware of? David speaks of God saying, "Your eyes saw my substance, being yet unformed. And in Your book they all were written, the days fashioned for me, when as yet there were none of them."[72] We see here that God knows the future. He knows everything that will ever happen to us. On the cross, Jesus didn't just make a blanket of forgiveness to throw over all of our sins. He suffered under the guilt and condemnation and

---

[72] Psalm 139:16

shame of each and every sin that each and every one of us have and ever will commit.

Knowing everything that I would ever do, He accepted me as His child. That means that nothing will ever come up in the future that will ever make God say, "Oops! I didn't account for that. I forgot to pay for that one on the cross. I guess you're on your own now." No, that will never happen! It doesn't matter what I do, Jesus has already paid the price for it on the cross. He offers me His forgiveness full and free. Why wouldn't He? He already paid the price!

But just because He paid the price for your sin and mine, doesn't mean that we are automatically forgiven. There are always two sides to the equation.

God's grace provided for the forgiveness, but it is our exercise of faith that accepts the forgiveness so that it becomes ours. And faith complies with the conditions of forgiveness.

The Steps of Forgiveness

To understand this a little more, let us look at the steps of forgiveness.

1. The Plan of Salvation.

Before we were even aware of our need of it, God put into place the whole plan of salvation to save us from the impossible mess we got ourselves into. Christ is "the Lamb slain from the foundation of the world."[73] He came "to seek and to save that which was lost."[74] And He couldn't wait until we were better to save us. He had to save us in the condition we were in. "But God demonstrates His own love toward us, in that while we were still sinners, Christ died for us."[75]

---

[73] Revelation 13:8
[74] Luke 19:10
[75] Romans 5:8

2. Working of the Holy Spirit

God always makes the first move. Men only respond to what God is already doing in the life. Human nature is such that we have no desire for righteousness. We naturally see no problem with sin. We gravitate toward it naturally. "The carnal mind is enmity against God; for it is not subject to the law of God, nor indeed can be."[76]

But God has sent His Holy Spirit to work upon our hearts and minds so that we might even desire forgiveness, restoration, and righteousness. "It is God who works in you both to will and to do for His good pleasure."[77] When we have a desire to be righteous, forgiven, and restored from our current state, it is evidence that God is *already* working in our lives to save us.

3. Conviction of Sin

The working of the Holy Spirit in my life brings me to the law of God and shows me that I am a sinner. "Whosoever committeth sin transgresseth also the law: for sin is the transgression of the law."[78] "By the law is the knowledge of sin."[79] As the law of God is revealed to me as the great standard by which all men will be judged, and as I see that I fall far short of this standard, I am convicted that I am a sinner. ""For I acknowledge my transgressions, and my sin is always before me."[80] Therefore, I recognize that I need a Savior.

4. Cooperation of the Will

Now that I am convicted that I am a sinner in need of a Savior, I must enlist my will to act upon those convictions and choose whom I will serve. "Choose for yourselves this day whom you will serve."[81] Will I continue to serve self, or will I surrender what I want to what

---

[76] Romans 8:7
[77] Philippians 2:13
[78] 1 John 3:4 KJV
[79] Romans 3:20
[80] Psalm 51:3
[81] Joshua 24:15

God wants and make a complete and total surrender of myself to Him? The will must be enlisted to make this decision and carry it into action.

5. Choose to Fulfill the Conditions of Forgiveness

The conditions of forgiveness include confession, repentance, and restoration.

Confession specifically acknowledges what was done or said and admits that it was wrong. In confession, I offer no excuse for why I did what I did. I only acknowledge that it was wrong. I seek forgiveness and restoration, even as I offer, to the best of my ability, proper restitution. "If we confess our sins, He is faithful and just to forgive us our sins and to cleanse us from all unrighteousness."[82]

Confession should be as broad as was the offence. If the sin is private, my confession should be to God only. If it affected my spouse, I should confess to them and to God. If it affected my whole family, I should confess to my whole family and to God. And if it affected my whole church, business, etc., then I should confess to my whole church, business, etc. and to God.

I had the opportunity of doing this not too long ago. A character defect that I possessed since childhood, but of which I was unaware, became apparent in a situation that arose in my church. When I became aware of this character defect, and when I saw how it had affected others at church, I realized that I needed to confess and apologize to the whole church.

So, the following weekend, I stood in front of the whole church and confessed my wrong and asked them to forgive me, and I promised that I would work on this defect with the Lord and, by God's grace, resolve this issue. It was embarrassing and humiliating, but it needed to be done, because I had hurt others and had spread a wrong influence through my behavior, and it needed to be corrected

---

[82] 1 John 1:9

so that negative influence would not continue to spread and hurt others.

Repentance involves sorrow for sin and a turning away from it. But repentance is not something that you and I produce. It is a gift of God. We cannot grunt, strain, moan, push, pull, or do anything hard enough to create repentance. We can simply ask for it and accept it by faith. And as the repentance becomes ours, we become sorry, not because we were caught, but because we disrespect, dishonor, misrepresent, and crucify again our Savior. We are not sorry because of the consequences that come to us because of the sin. We are sorry because of what we have done to God because of our sin. And as the repentance becomes ours, we exercise it in turning away from the thing we are repenting from. "He who covers his sins will not prosper, but whoever confesses and forsakes them will have mercy."[83]

Restoration involves giving back whatever is possible and appropriate in relation to a wrong. For example, an acquaintance of mine stole a sweater from a department store when he was young. A couple decades later, as conviction came upon him, he realized that he needed to restore what he stole. So, he went back to that department store and spoke with the manager and offered to pay for the sweater (at a current cost) with interest to cover what the store could have gained by investing that money over the last couple decades.

We are told, "Therefore if you bring your gift to the altar, and there remember that your brother has something against you, leave your gift there before the altar, and go your way. First be reconciled to your brother, and then come and offer your gift."[84] "If the wicked restores the pledge, gives back what he has stolen, and walks in the statutes of life without committing iniquity, he shall surely live; he shall not die."[85]

---

[83] Proverbs 28:13
[84] Matthew 5:23,24
[85] Ezekiel 33:15

6. *Believe & Accept the Divine Exchange at the Cross*

As we accept the divine exchange at the cross and enter into the life of Christ, we are empowered to overcome and set free from the past. "For God so loved the world that He gave His only begotten Son, that whoever believes in Him should not perish but have everlasting life." [86] We comply with the conditions above, and forgiveness and its sweet peace and joy are ours! I want that freedom, don't you?

The Results of Forgiveness

So, what are the results of forgiveness? I have no more guilt, even though I still remember what I did. I have no more bitterness, because they no longer did it to me. I love them because God loves them, and I want them to go free just like He set me free. And I will cooperate with the Holy Spirit in assisting in their freedom, even if it requires self-sacrifice.

What is one of the functions of forgiveness? It is to allow one to enter back into relationship with another. God wants a relationship with each of us, and His forgiveness is offered to each of us to allow us to enter back into relationship with Him. The cross makes this restoration of relationship possible. What amazing love! What great grace! What full forgiveness that flows from the heart of God toward us!

Take Up Our Cross

Because of what Jesus has done for you and me, we are gratefully indebted to Him. We love Him because of the freedom He has given to us, and our greatest joy is to obey and serve Him. And He bids us, "Whoever desires to come after Me, let him deny

---

[86] John 3:16

The Law of Life

himself, and take up his cross, and follow Me."[87] What does it mean to take up your cross and follow Jesus?

"Man is to leave the error of his ways, to follow the example of Christ, to take up his cross and follow Him, denying self, and obeying God at any cost."[88] "...to lift the cross...means to take up the very duties that cut across the natural appetites and passions."[89]

"True religion is the imitation of Christ. Those who follow Christ will deny self, take up the cross, and walk in His footsteps. Following Christ means obedience to all His commandments. No soldier can be said to follow his commander unless he obeys orders. Christ if our model. To copy Jesus, full of love and tenderness and compassion, will require that we draw near to Him daily."[90]

"He says to us, 'If any man will come after me, let him deny himself, and take up his cross daily, and follow me.' Christ alone can make us capable of responding when He says, 'Take my yoke upon you, and learn of me; for I am meek and lowly in heart.' This means that every day self must be denied. Christ can give us the noble resolve, the will to suffer, and to fight the battles of the Lord with persevering energy. The weakest, aided by divine grace, may have strength to be more than conqueror."[91]

Toward the end of this book, you will see what taking up your cross really means and what it looks like. When that key ingredient is in your life, all of what was mentioned already in taking up your cross and following Jesus will become a joyful and natural part of your life.

---

[87] Mark 8:34
[88] White, E. G. (1991) *Counsels for the Church.* (p 269). Nampa, ID: Pacific Press Publishing Association.
[89] White, E. G. (1875) *Testimonies for the Church, Volume 3.* (p 63). Mountain View, CA: Pacific Press Publishing Association.
[90] White, E. G. (1957) *S.D.A. Bible Commentary Volume 7.* (p 949). Washington, D.C.: Review and Herald Publishing Association.
[91] White, E. G. (1976) *Maranatha.* (p 85). Washington, D.C.: Review and Herald Publishing Association.

The Law of Life

CHAPTER SEVEN

The Talent of Suffering

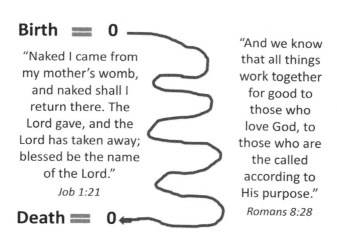

Birth = 0

"Naked I came from my mother's womb, and naked shall I return there. The Lord gave, and the Lord has taken away; blessed be the name of the Lord."

Job 1:21

Death = 0

"And we know that all things work together for good to those who love God, to those who are the called according to His purpose."

Romans 8:28

Losing Loved Ones

I want to switch topics slightly and look at loss from another perspective. I have talked with many individuals who have developed cancer and other serious health conditions, and when I explore their life and experiences prior to developing their health challenge, I frequently find that they have lost a significant loved one in the years prior to their illness. But there are others who lose loved ones and do just fine. What is the difference? Does the Bible give us the correct perspective on how to deal with the loss of loved ones? It does.

At birth, how much do we have? How much do we possess? Absolutely nothing. At death, how much will we have? Absolutely nothing.

Between birth and death there is this squiggly line called life. Life has ups and downs, its good times and not so good times. We meet people, we learn to love people, and we lose people in this path. If I start this pathway with nothing, and I finish this pathway with nothing, then is everything between point B (birth) and Point D (death) a gain or a loss?

Job gives us a good perspective on this topic. After losing all of his children, his animals, and his servants in one day, Job says. "Naked I came from my mother's womb, and naked shall I return there. The Lord gave, and the Lord has taken away; blessed be the name of the Lord."[92] Job recognized that he began his journey of life without anything, and he would end his journey without anything, so anything that he had between point B & point D was a gain.

When you start and end without anything, when everything you have is not yours but the Lord's, when you didn't produce it, and when you are not even your own, you can't lose anything.

Imagine that you are the steward of a wealthy businessman's estate. Your job is to keep everything in good repair and operating smoothly. The owner has seven Lamborghinis that you help maintain. One day, the owner decides to give away two of the Lamborghinis. Now you are only steward of five Lamborghinis. Do you get upset at the owner because you lost two Lamborghinis? No. That would be ridiculous. They weren't yours. They were the owner's. He can get rid of them whenever he wants to.

---

[92] Job 1:21

God is the owner, but we go through life like we are the owners. If the car is stolen, I get all upset, because I think it was my car. If the house burns down, I mourn the loss, as if it was mine, but it was never mine. It all belongs to God. He is the owner. We are just the stewards.

Remember the family who lost their 11-year-old daughter? If they mourn like people normally mourn, it will break down their constitutions and some physical problem will develop in their bodies later. How would they mourn?

They might have thoughts like this, "She was only 11 years old. She missed out on so much. We won't be able to see her graduate from elementary school, high school, or college. We won't be able to walk her down the aisle and see her married. We won't have the joy of grandchildren from her." And so on. What are they mourning for? They are mourning for that which they never had. They never had tomorrow. They never had the graduations. They never had the son-in-law or the grandchildren. What they mourn is the loss of that which they expect. Were they ever guaranteed tomorrow? No. They only have now.

Those parents could either live the rest of their lives in loss, mourning the cruel death of their 11-year-old daughter, or they could live a life of gratitude, thankful for the 11 years of life they had with their daughter. Was their experience a loss or was it a gain? Did they have her when they were born? No. Would they have her when they died? No. So, even though she died, they are not at loss. They are actually in gain, because they had 11 years with her. They were blessed with 11 years of smiles, hugs, shared experiences, and companionship. They were blessed with 11 years!

If their perspective is one of gratitude for how God blessed them with 11 years with that daughter, if they focused on what they had gained rather than what they had supposedly lost, if they had remembered that they were only the steward and not the owner, how would their health be after the death of their daughter? It would remain good.

I am not trying to say that it is wrong or a sin to mourn. I am not saying that at all. What I am saying is that when we have the correct perspective, we will get to the point where we won't *have to* mourn in the usual way that people mourn. And with the correct perspective, our thoughts will not cause dysfunction in the body as happens when our thoughts are wrong.

Paul gives us a better perspective on this issue when he says, "And we know that all things work together for good to those who love God, to those who are the called according to His purpose."[93] What Paul is telling us is that God can take whatever comes our way and turn it into good. Even the things that seem like the most difficult and impossible to endure are talents that God can use for good. He doesn't allow anything to befall us that He doesn't plan to use for our good and for the good of others.

The following is one of my favorite quotes. "The Father's presence encircled Christ, and nothing befell Him but that which infinite love permitted for the blessing of the world. Here was His source of comfort, and it is for us. He who is imbued with the Spirit of Christ abides in Christ. The blow that is aimed at him falls upon the Saviour, who surrounds him with His presence. Whatever comes to him comes from Christ. He has no need to resist evil, for Christ is his defense. Nothing can touch him except by our Lord's permission, and 'all things' that are permitted 'work together for good to them that love God.' Romans 8:28."[94]

What this quote tells me is that God surrounds every one of His children with His own presence. If someone comes up to me to punch me in the face, their fist must go through God first in order to get to me. And God will only allow that fist to get through if He can

[93] Romans 8:28
[94] White, E. G. (1896) *Thoughts from the Mount of Blessing.* (p 71). Mountain View, CA: Pacific Press Publishing Association.

work it out for good. I don't have to defend myself. God is my defense. I can turn the other cheek.

There is another promise in 1 Corinthians 10:13 that tells us that God will not allow us to be tempted beyond what we are able, but with the temptation will also make the way of escape. That means that God won't allow anything to come to us unless He will give us strength to endure. That means that anything that comes to us, no matter how bad it may be, is wrapped with God's love, assuring us that it will work out for good, and He will give us strength to endure. What a merciful God we serve! We can trust Him even with the most painful circumstances and experiences of our lives.

The Talent of Suffering

A talent is defined as a natural ability, an endowment, or an aptitude. We usually think of talents in relation to someone's capacity to excel in doing something. But did you realize that suffering can be a talent? It can be an endowed ability or aptitude that can be used for good. And just like the other talents Jesus talked about, if this talent is buried, God cannot be glorified through it. He is robbed of His purpose through allowing it. But if it is used, God is glorified. Are you using your talent of suffering? Or is it buried, lost to the world, useless in its unused state?

Before I go further, I want to clarify something. God is not the author of suffering. Suffering is a result of sin—of choosing to separate from God and sever our ties with the Source of life. Suffering is the result of the working of an enemy. Peter tells us, "Be sober, be vigilant; because your adversary the devil walks about like a roaring lion, seeking whom he may devour."[95]

And Jesus tells us, "The thief does not come except to steal, and to kill, and to destroy. I have come that they may have life, and that

---

[95] 1 Peter 5:8

they may have it more abundantly."[96] Again, God is not the cause or author of suffering. Suffering is the result of the work of an enemy.

And God is the master of weaving His goodness and love through all of the tangled mess of pain and suffering that the devil causes so that He can rescue His children from the enemy and then make them instruments in the salvation of others.

So, let us consider a little closer the topic of suffering and how it can be a talent.

Who can best comfort a mother who has lost her new-born child? Another mother who has lost her new-born child and made it through. Who can best comfort someone who lost their leg? Someone else who lost their leg and have overcome their disability. Who can best comfort someone struggling with a challenging disease? Someone else who has gone through the same struggling disease and has survived and thrived.

How can suffering be a talent? Satan hates God and wants nothing more than to hurt Him. And Satan knows that the best way to hurt God is to hurt His children, as God experiences and identifies with everything His children go through. Everyone is God's child, so, God has children who are suffering from all types of issues and in all types of situations around the world. And God wants to reach those who are suffering and comfort them. But God needs others who understand what it is like to go through the pain and suffering to best comfort those who are currently in the pain and suffering. God needs others who can reach His other children who are going through the same thing.

"In God's great plan for the redemption of a lost race, He has placed Himself under the necessity of using human agencies as His helping hand. He must have a helping hand, in order to reach humanity. He must have the cooperation of those who will be active,

---

quick to see opportunities, quick to discern what must be done for their fellow men."[97]

The proper use of the talent of suffering is going up to someone who is suffering from the same thing Satan brought you through and God rescued you from, and saying, "I know what you are going through. I've been there too, and God got me through it. Let me tell you how I made it through."

But if you bury your talent, God's purpose in bringing you through your suffering and turning it into good will be thwarted. And that child of His who is suffering, whom you could help, may never be reached by His love in the way that God designed they should be reached.

In the early 1900's a passenger train derailed near Chicago. Hundreds were killed or injured in the accident, but in one of the rear passenger cars which had not derailed, there was a red cross nurse. As she worked her way up the wreckage, assisting whomever she could, she looked over and saw a well-dressed man looking at all of the injured passengers. Recognizing that he was a well-known Chicago surgeon, she went over to him, and shook him out of his daze to ask him to help her care for the injured. As he was coming out of his dazed state, he said to her, "My instruments!" And then he went about helping whomever he could.

Later that evening, the two of them met again, and as he thanked her for taking the lead in helping the wounded, she was curious and asked him, "When I found you, you were just standing there, not doing anything. And when I got your attention, you said, 'My instruments.' What was going on?"

He replied, "I was standing there looking at all of these injured people and thinking to myself, 'My instruments, my instruments, if only I had my surgical instruments, I could help them.' You see, I am a surgeon, and I do what I do well, but I need my instruments in

---

[97] White, E.G. (1958) *Selected Messages Book 1.* (p. 99). Washington, D.C.: Review and Herald Publishing Association.

order to do what I do. I didn't have my instruments with me, so I could do very little for them."

God is the master surgeon, but He has pledged himself to use human beings to reach human beings. He has His children in all forms of suffering, and He needs other children trained by those same experiences in suffering to reach those who are going through those same trials. Those of us who have suffered are His instruments to reach others who are similarly suffering.

What instrument can the surgeon use best? It is the one he can use in the most situations and circumstances. I want to encourage you by one other thought. The more you have suffered, the more useful you are as an instrument in God's hands, because you can identify with more people in their suffering. You can look at more people in the eye and honestly tell them, "I know what you are going through. I have been there too. Let me tell you how God got me through."

Do you want heaven's perspective on suffering? Here it is. "God never leads His children otherwise than they would choose to be led, if they could see the end from the beginning, and discern the glory of the purpose which they are fulfilling as co-workers with Him. Not Enoch, who was translated to heaven, not Elijah, who ascended in a chariot of fire, was greater or more honored than John the Baptist, who perished alone in the dungeon. "Unto you it is given in the behalf of Christ, not only to believe on Him, but also to suffer for His sake." Philippians 1:29. And of all the gifts that Heaven can bestow upon men, fellowship with Christ in His sufferings is the most weighty trust and the highest honor."[98]

Rather than being a curse, or something to be looked down upon, fellowship with Christ in His sufferings is the most weighty trust and the highest honor. It is the most honorable gift heaven can bestow upon you.

---

[98] White, E. G. (1898). *The Desire of Ages.* (p 224). Mountain View, CA: Pacific Press Publishing Association.

And there is another purpose for suffering that we must consider. In the context of sin, suffering is a necessary part of molding us into the image of Christ. The diamond can never become a diamond without extreme pressure and heat, but the beauty and worth of the diamond are worth all of the pressure and heat that is necessary in its formation. God sees us as His precious jewels, not worthless coal, and so He permits the pressure and heat to come so that we can become precious jewels that we become beautiful, reflecting His love and character to others.

"We are forming characters for heaven. No character can be complete without trial and suffering. We must be tested, we must be tried. Christ bore the test of character in our behalf that we might bear this test in our own behalf through the divine strength He has brought to us."[99]

"Many who sincerely consecrate their lives to God's service are surprised and disappointed to find themselves, as never before, confronted by obstacles and beset by trials and perplexities. They pray for Christlikeness of character, for a fitness for the Lord's work, and they are placed in circumstances that seem to call forth all the evil of their nature. Faults are revealed of which they did not even suspect the existence. Like Israel of old they question, 'If God is leading us, why do all these things come upon us?'

It is because God is leading them that these things come upon them. Trials and obstacles are the Lord's chosen methods of discipline and His appointed conditions of success. He who reads the hearts of men knows their characters better than they themselves know them. He sees that some have powers and susceptibilities which, rightly directed, might be used in the advancement of His work.

---

[99] White, EG. (1979). *This Day With God*. (p 427). Washington, D.C.: Review and Herald Publishing Association.

In His providence He brings these persons into different positions and varied circumstances that they may discover in their character the defects which have been concealed from their own knowledge. He gives them opportunity to correct these defects and to fit themselves for His service. Often, He permits the fires of affliction to assail them that they may be purified.

The fact that we are called upon to endure trial shows that the Lord Jesus sees in us something precious which He desires to develop. If He saw in us nothing whereby He might glorify His name, He would not spend time in refining us. He does not cast worthless stones into His furnace. It is valuable ore that He refines.

The blacksmith puts the iron and steel into the fire that he may know what manner of metal they are. The Lord allows His chosen ones to be placed in the furnace of affliction to prove what temper they are of and whether they can be fashioned for His work. The potter takes the clay and molds it according to his will. He kneads it and works it. He tears it apart and presses it together. He wets it and then dries it. He lets it lie for a while without touching it. When it is perfectly pliable, he continues the work of making of it a vessel.

He forms it into shape and on the wheel trims and polishes it. He dries it in the sun and bakes it in the oven. Thus it becomes a vessel fit for use. So the great Master Worker desires to mold and fashion us. And as the clay is in the hands of the potter, so are we to be in His hands. We are not to try to do the work of the potter. Our part is to yield ourselves to be molded by the Master Worker."[100]

Peter admonishes us, "Beloved, think it not strange concerning the fiery trial which is to try you, as though some strange thing happened unto you: but rejoice, inasmuch as ye are partakers of Christ's sufferings; that, when His glory shall be revealed, ye may be glad also with exceeding joy."[101]

---

[100] White, E.G. (1905) The Ministry of Healing. (pp. 469-471). Mountain View, CA: Pacific Press Publishing Association.
[101] 1 Peter 4:12,13

Who Can Hurt Me?

Now let's look back at the topic of the heart and personal hurts. Who can hurt me? From an emotional or spiritual standpoint, no one can hurt me, I can only hurt myself. You see, only I can breathe for myself. Only I can eat for myself. Only I can drink for myself. And only I can think for myself. Only MY breathing, eating, and drinking—not somebody else's—impacts my body & my health. Only my thinking impacts my body & my health.

What someone else does may provide a hurtful environment from which I could feed from, but the buffet of God's love is always present, so I will never be in a situation where I *must* choose from the hurtful environment that "they" provide. I have a choice, and I can choose from the buffet of God's love. It is my option whether to think hurtful thoughts or loving thoughts. I have the power to do the one or the other. It is my own decisions, my own thinking—not their actions—that determines my outcome.

Patient Examples
Martha

Herb and Martha had been married for 35 years. Herb was a traveling salesman, and Martha was a homemaker. Herb was gone to work during the week and home on the weekends. Their marriage was fairly good as far as marriages go, not too great, not too poor. That is...until Martha found out.

She found out that Herb was not exactly faithful to her. In fact, she found out that he had been unfaithful to her for the entire 35 years of their marriage. In fact, she found out that he had another family in another city, whom he lived with during the week, and she was his second wife!

During the three years following this discovery, Martha's health began to decline rapidly. It seemed as though one health challenge followed the other until her situation appeared to be hopeless.

What was the cause of Martha's decline? Was it her husband's infidelity? No! He had been cheating on her for 35 years, and it didn't affect her one bit. She didn't become sick until she *knew* what was going on. The cause of Martha's decline was not his infidelity. It was her thinking. You see, she thought he was hers, she thought she loved him with her love, he was her love source, and she was in significant personal loss because of this. But was he hers? Was it her love? Was he really the source of her love? No. Did she really have anything to lose? No. She could have looked at the situation and been grateful for how he had supported her over the years. She could have been thankful to God for supporting her all these years. She could have celebrated the good weekends they had for 35 years. And if she would have done that, what would her health have been like now?

It was not what happened to her that destroyed her health. It was her thinking about what happened to her that destroyed her health. I see this all the time in my practice. I see people who develop cancer in times of great loss. I see people with autoimmune disorders following great losses. I see people physically all messed up because of personal loss.

At this point, someone in a similar situation usually will ask the painful question, "Do you mean my disease is my fault?" And my answer is, "Yes, it is your fault." But I am quick to follow with this observation: if it is someone else's fault—if someone else is the cause— then you can't do anything about it. You are stuck with no solutions, because you can't fix or change them. But if you are the one at fault, there is hope, because God, with your cooperation, can fix the problem. If you are at fault, there is hope!

When I give the gift of time or love or concern or care, I can recognize that I am just the delivery guy. I am just the steward of God's resources, and if I am rejected, it is not me who is rejected, because I am God's. He is the one rejected. If the gift is destroyed, it was God's gift, not mine. If the car is stolen, it was God's car, not mine. I don't have to be upset and hurt, because it's not mine. It's God's.

Taking It Personally

From another perspective, many of our problems come because we take things personally. Imagine that your cat is playing on the table, knocks over a glass, and water spills all over the table. Why is it that there is *water* all over the table? If you bump into the table and the glass spills over and there is coffee all over the table, why is it that there is *coffee* all over the table? If an earthquake comes along and the glass on the table spills over and there is milk all over the table, why is it that there is *milk* all over the table? And if you are carrying a glass and you trip and wine spills all over the carpet, why is it that there is *wine* all over the carpet?

You might say that water is on the table because the cat knocked over the glass, coffee is on the table because you bumped into the table, milk is on the table because of the shaking of the earthquake, and wine is all over the floor because you tripped. But what if I said that all of the glasses were empty? What would you blame now?

The reality is that what is on the table or on the carpet is there because that is what was in the glass before it was spilled over. If there was nothing in the glass before it was turned over, nothing could come out. Water came out because water was in there. Water couldn't come out if water wasn't in there. Coffee came out because coffee was in there. Coffee couldn't come out if coffee wasn't in there. The same is true of people.

If someone says something to you that is hurtful, it has nothing to do with you. It has everything to do with them. Why? Because it couldn't come out of them if it were not in them. Just like the cup that is spilled over. It doesn't matter what it was that spilled the cup over, what comes out comes out because it was in there. The same is true of people. It doesn't matter what triggers them to say what they do and act the way they do; whatever they say, however they say it, and whatever they do comes out of them because it was in them.

The Bible, in Luke 6:45 says, "For out of the abundance of the heart the mouth speaks." And Proverbs 4:23 tells us, "Keep your heart with all diligence, for out of it spring the issues of life." What the Bible is telling us is that what someone else says or does to us is not about us. It is about them. Because it could not come out of them if it were not in them. So, don't take personally what others say and do to you. It really has nothing to do with you. It has everything to do with them.

That being said, it is possible that they are telling the truth, so it behooves each of us to pay attention to what is being said and bring it in prayer to the Lord and compare it with the Bible to see if what they are saying is true. I may need to change what I do and how I do it, because it is affecting others negatively.

The opposite is also true. It doesn't matter what someone else does or says. It doesn't matter what your circumstances are. It doesn't matter how tired you are or how stressed or pressured you are. Your response—what comes out of you—has nothing to do with them or your circumstances. Your response could not come out unless it were in you—in your heart. Your response reveals to you what is truly in your heart, "For out of the abundance of the heart the mouth speaks."

So, in an argument or stressful situations, watch yourself, not them, and see what is coming out of you, for that reveals what is in you. Then go to work with God to resolve those things that are revealed.

Margaret

Margaret came to see a colleague of mine a few years ago. She had been coughing uncontrollably for a couple years, and she also suffered from urinary incontinence—unable to hold her urine in for more than 30 minutes or when she was coughing. She had seen many doctors and tried many treatments, all without success. She came to see my colleague to see if he could identify the cause of her coughing, and after examining her, he did not find a source. But he asked her about her life and about love issues.

What he discovered was that Margaret had been in a prolonged conflict with her daughter over her daughter's boyfriend. Margaret didn't like the boyfriend, and her daughter wouldn't listen to Margaret regarding the relationship. Margaret, as many parents do, tried to control her daughter, and her daughter had been in rebellion for several years, leaving home and moving in with the boyfriend. My colleague talked with Margaret about the Law of Life, and encouraged her to come to God every morning, so that she could take of His love. He instructed her to see how much God loves her daughter and has forgiven her, and to forgive her likewise.

He talked with her about principles of love and freedom and encouraged her to stop trying to control her daughter, and simply to love her. And he challenged her to practice only thinking positive thoughts about her daughter and the boyfriend. When Margaret returned to his office a few weeks later, she was no longer coughing, and her urinary incontinence was resolved!

So, was it all just in her head? No! There were very real physical things going on in her body. But the foundation of the issue was in her mind. The conflict with her daughter, and her attempt to control her (which, by the way, is not what love does), was the foundation of her chronic cough and urinary incontinence. Once the cause was removed, the effect ceased.

Janet

Janet suffered from severe migraine headaches. They started 13 years before and recurred every weekend. She would be fine through the week, but they would begin on Friday and continue through Monday morning. She frequently received medications, injections, and IV fluids, because she would keep vomiting and could not keep anything down. She had gone from doctor to doctor, trying to find a solution to her issues, but without success. Then one day, she went to see my colleague. After examining her and reviewing her medical record and not finding anything physical to explain her symptoms, he began to ask about her past.

She related to him that her father was an alcoholic and was mean when he was drunk. He worked in another city, and was away from the home during the week, but would come home on Friday, stay for the weekend, and head back to work on Monday morning. She hated her father and how he treated her. Several months before her migraines began, her father died. My colleague immediately saw the correlation between her father's presence in the home on weekends, and Janet's pattern of migraines on weekends. He shared with her the Law of Life, and encouraged her to spend time every morning with God, taking of the love He offered.

He encouraged her to see her father through God's eyes of love, and to ask God to give her a heart to love her father. He challenged her to think only positive thoughts about him and to forgive him. Janet began putting these things into practice, and within a week she stopped having migraine headaches.

So, was it all just in her head? No! There were very real physical things going on in her body. But the foundation of the issue was in her mind. Her hatred for her father (which, by the way, is not what love does), was the foundation of her migraine headaches. Once the cause was removed, the effect ceased.

Carl

Carl was a 65 y/o diabetic cattle rancher in Idaho. One day, he noticed an ulcer on his foot, and he immediately went to his doctor to check it out. He was placed on a course of antibiotics, and when he returned, it wasn't any better, so his doctor debrided the ulcer (that means he cut out the dead tissue) and put him on another course of antibiotics. His sugars were not under control, so they were working on medications and lifestyle changes, but he didn't improve. Eventually, infection got to the bone, and Carl was sent to the surgeon.

The surgeon told him he needed to amputate his little toe in order to save the rest of the foot. After the amputation, Carl was sent to see a diabetes specialist, who worked with him on his sugars. Despite the help of the diabetes specialist, his sugars still weren't under control. His wound got worse and infected the bone of the next toe, and again, he saw the surgeon for another amputation. Two toes down, three to go, but you can't handle weight on the foot if you have too few toes, so the next amputation would be across the middle of the foot.

His diabetes specialist admitted him to the ICU so that they could put him on an insulin drip and see if they could get his sugars under control, and even in the ICU on an insulin drip they couldn't get his sugars under control.

So, he is seeing his surgeon again, who is completely confused. No one can figure out what is going on. His foot wound is getting worse and he will soon need another amputation. So, the surgeon tells Carl about a new physician in town who does things a little differently. John, another colleague of mine, is an internal medicine specialist with a strong interest in lifestyle. In fact, he and his family ran a lifestyle program in their home for a while. Anyway, Carl gets referred to John.

When John sees Carl, he reviews his medical information and looks through all of his doctor's notes, x-rays and MRI scans, and talks with Carl about his lifestyle and diet, etc. In all of this, John can't find anything significant that Carl isn't already complying with. But

John has a questionnaire that he gives to each of his patients, and the questionnaire asks about grief, anxiety, discontent, remorse, guilt, and distrust. It also asks about courage, hope, faith, sympathy, and love. And on that questionnaire, one result was very abnormal. Carl was dealing with a lot of guilt.

When asked about the guilt, Carl mentioned that he was a Christian, and he knew that he should be taking care of his body, but he obviously hadn't done a good job at doing that, and he felt guilty because he was responsible for the health problems he was facing. John asked Carl, "In your church, what do you do when you feel guilty about something?

Carl said, "Well, we pray and ask God to forgive us." John said, "Well, what about praying now?" Then and there in the office, Carl knelt down and prayed and asked God to forgive him for not taking care of his body like he was supposed to. After getting up off his knees and sitting back in the chair, John asked Carl, "In your church, after you pray and ask God to forgive you, what do you do?" Carl said, "Well, we trust that God forgave us, and we don't do the bad things any more. But Doc, I'm already not doing those things anymore." John could not identify anything else to address, Carl left, and John felt somewhat dissatisfied with the whole encounter, because he didn't feel like he had helped Carl that much.

But after that meeting, Carl's blood sugars started to be controlled, his foot started to heal, and within 6 weeks his foot had healed up, after 4 months of doctors, hospitals, medications, surgeries, and ICU stays. The only issue that was identified and addressed was guilt.

So, was it all just in his head? No! There were very real physical things going on in his body. But the foundation of the issue was in his mind. His guilt (which, by the way, is not what love allows), was the foundation of his diabetic foot ulcer. Once the cause was removed, the effect ceased.

Michelle

I took care of Michelle several years ago, when she came to our lifestyle center with cancer. She had multiple tumors in her abdomen, and she had already failed several chemotherapy attempts. So, she came looking for another way to help herself be healthy. We do not cure cancer. We simply teach people how to live the healthiest way possible within the context of their disease to give them the best chance of healing.

As I met with Michelle, it became evident that there were some issues going on in her life that were not helping her cancer. We helped her correct some of her lifestyle issues and used some simple remedies to help her out. But the big issue, as I met and counselled with her, was her issue with her mother.

Michelle never knew her father. Her mother raised her for a few years and then left Michelle with her grandparents for them to raise her. Michelle's mother would come back into her life periodically, and thoughts and feelings of resentment, abandonment, anger, confusion, etc. would well up in Michelle. It was evident that she didn't love and honor her mother, and I knew that couldn't be good for her cancer.

So, I counselled with Michelle, helping her to see that her mother is not her source. God is. I challenged her to go to God and take of His perfect love and ask Him to give her the same love for her mother. I helped Michelle to see that she doesn't have to take what her mother does personally, because what her mother does is not about Michelle. It is about her mother, because what comes out of her mother does so because that is what is inside of her.

Michelle took this to heart and began spending time alone with God and learning to take from Him so that she could love her mother with God's love.

Before Michelle came to our center, her cancer markers were elevated, but two weeks later, they were back into the normal range. A couple months later we received a happy report that nearly half of her tumors were gone, and the remaining ones were smaller than before.

But about four months after that, I received a report that Michelle was discouraged, because her cancer marker tests were back up again. So, I called her and found out that her mother had come back into the picture and stirred things all up again. Michelle forgot much of what I had taught her, and she was back to taking things personally and seeing her mother as her source. So, we spent another hour going over the principles again and helping her regain a correct perspective. She did. And a couple months later, we had the joyful report that her cancer markers were back down into the normal range.

So, was it all just in her head? No! There was very real cancer in her body. But the foundation of the cancer was in her mind. Her resentment toward her mother (which, by the way, is not what love does), was the foundation of her cancer. Once the cause was removed, the effect ceased. When the cause returned, the effect returned as well.

You see, most of our diseases have their foundation in the mind. "Sickness of the mind prevails everywhere. Nine tenths of the diseases from which men suffer have their foundation here."[102]

Now, I don't want you to get the idea that everything—all disease—has its foundation in the mind. But I do want you to recognize that most of it does. Ninety percent of it, to be exact.

---

[102] White, E. G. (1923) *Counsels on Health*. (p 324). Mountain View, CA: Pacific Press Publishing Association.

CHAPTER EIGHT

The Law of Love...and Health

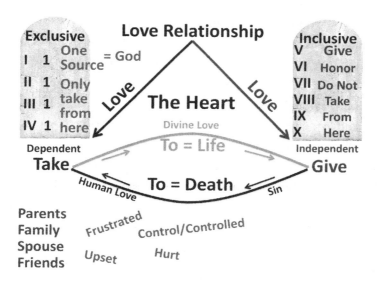

Love and the Law

L et us take one more look at love relationships and their impact on health. There are two legitimate love relationships that function in the heart. The one love relationship is a relationship from which I take. The other love relationship is a relationship to which I give. Both are legitimate love relationships. And God has created us so that we take from one relationship in order to give to another. This is how divine love functions in the redeemed heart.

But the enemy, who cannot create anything new, has messed up God's plan by simply turning the equation around. Instead of taking to give, we then give to take (receive), going in the opposite direction that God designed for us—making a "new order" of things according to Satan's way. This "new order" is found in human love, which resulted because of sin. Now, to follow God's design brings life, but following the enemy's plan brings death.

Have you ever wondered why God wrote the ten commandments on two tables of stone? When I was young, I guess I just thought it was because His finger was too big to write everything on one stone. But that is not the case. He had a purpose in writing the commandments on two stones.

You see, each table of the commandments governs each of the love relationships. The first four commandments are exclusive commands, and the last six are inclusive commands. According to the first commandment, how many gods are there? One and only One. And the second commandment states that we are to worship how many gods? One and only One. And the third commandment states that we are to reverence and make holy the name of how many? One and only One. And the fourth commandment states that we are to worship specifically on how many days of the week? One and only One. The first four commandments are exclusive, meaning that they include only one, and exclude all else.

In essence, what the first four commandments are saying is: there is only one source, and that source is God. Another way of putting it is this: *Only take from here.* These four commandments govern the exclusive taking love relationship. We are to take from God as our only source.

But what about the other six commandments? The fifth commandment states that we are to do what to our parents? We are to honor them. To honor our parents—is that giving or is that taking? It is giving.

So, the next set of commandments govern the giving love. Does the fifth commandment give any qualifications of one's parents that would exclude them from this commandment? Does it say for you to honor your parents only if they are honorable? No! The commandment says to honor your parents, regardless of whether they are honorable or not. It is inclusive. It includes all parents, no matter what their qualifications or characteristics are. We are simply to give honor to them. But what about the other five commandments (You shall not murder...commit adultery...steal...bear false witness...covet)?

All of these commandments say, "Do not take from here!" It doesn't matter who they are, how they treat you, what they have, or how they look. You give to them. You don't take from them.

The one you take from, you are dependent upon. But the one that you give to, you are independent of.

For example, imagine a pure mountain stream flowing to the valley below, and along the stream there are three farms. You purchase the second farm, the one in the middle, and you are very happy with your situation. You use the water from the stream to provide water to your home, you use it to water your fields and keep your crops and animals alive, and you enjoy sitting by the crystal-clear stream in the afternoons.

Let us say that the neighbor downstream from you decides that they are going to start some kind of manufacturing industry, and they divert all of the water from the stream coming into their property to their manufacturing plant, and only a little, polluted water flows out of their farm downstream. Does their decision affect you directly? No!

Why? Because they are downstream from you. You still have access to all of the water that you need and can use it for what you need/want, and what they do with the water after that is their problem. You aren't dependent upon them, because they don't control your source.

But let us imagine that the neighbor upstream from you decides they are going to start the same manufacturing industry, and they divert all of the water from the stream to their manufacturing plant, and only a little, polluted water flows out of their farm to yours. Does their decision affect you directly? Yes! Why? Because they are upstream from you. You need the water that comes through their farm to your farm. They control your source, and so you are dependent upon them. And what they do directly affects you. If they are one you take from—if they are upstream from you, if they are your source—you are dependent upon them. But if they are the one you give to—if they are downstream from you, if they are not your source—you are independent of them. What they do doesn't affect or control you.

We find ourselves in a problem. You see, the law is not governing our lives, and we have everything backward. Instead of only having God as our source, our parents, our family, our spouses, our friends—and even our pets—are our sources.

How can you know if they are your source? You are dependent upon them. They frustrate you. They make you upset. They hurt you. And they try to control you, while you try to control them. You see, you have to control your sources if you can't fully trust them, because you have to protect yourself by protecting your sources. And you cannot trust any human being, so if they are your source, you must try to control them.

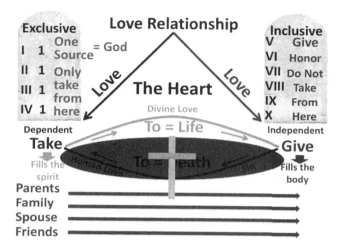

But God never intended for others to be your source (except for young children in their parents' care, which is temporary and should result in the parents weaning the children from them as a source to God as the source). The law states that God is our only source. Everyone else is there for us to give to, no matter who they are or what they are like.

Through the sacrifice that He made on the cross, and the working of the Holy Spirit in the heart, God wipes out the old heart of sin, with its giving to receive, and with its putting others in the place where only God should be, and He restores us to the heart of divine love which He created us to enjoy originally.

In giving us that new heart, God restores the function of the law in our hearts through the work of the Holy Spirit. "But this is the covenant that I will make with the house of Israel after those days, says the Lord: I will put My law in their minds, and write it on their hearts; and I will be their God, and they shall be My people." Jeremiah 31:33. And when the law is restored to its proper function in us, our parents will cease to be our source. Our family will cease to be our source. Our spouse will cease to be our source. Our friends and our pets will cease to be our source. Everyone will be someone whom we give to, not take from, and God will be our only source.

And when you and I take from God, that taking results in the filling of the spirit (from outside of itself - from God) with what it needs (love). And when you give to others, thought is converted to physical action like speaking and doing, and that giving fills the body (from the spirit) with what it needs (energy/power/control).

So, ultimately our problem is the sources we choose to take from. As long as I live by the law of God, taking love from God and giving love to others, I will have health. But if I start taking love from the wrong sources or keeping it to myself, I will eventually experience symptoms, disease, and eventually death. When that law that governs love is broken, that is called sin, and sin is the root cause of disease. It is interesting. When you read the Bible, and it talks about being healthy, it doesn't instruct you to eat your greens. It instructs you to obey the law.

"If you diligently heed the voice of the Lord your God and do what is right in His sight, give ear to His commandments and keep all His statutes, I will put none of the diseases on you which I have brought on the Egyptians. For I am the Lord who heals you."[103] Do you want health? Do you want to be free from the diseases of the Egyptians (they suffered from heart disease, cancer, diabetes, etc.)? Then "give ear to His commandments and keep all His statutes."

Do you want healthy skin and muscles, and strong bones? "Do not be wise in your own eyes; fear the Lord and depart from evil. It will be health to your flesh, and strength to your bones."[104]

Do you want life? "My son, give attention to my words; incline your ear to my sayings. Do not let them depart from your eyes; keep them in the midst of your heart; for they are life to those who find

---

[103] Exodus 15:26
[104] Proverbs 3:7,8

them, and health to all their flesh. Keep your heart with all diligence, for out of it spring the issues of life."[105]

Do you want to be blessed, fertile, and healthy? "Then it shall come to pass, because you listen to these judgments, and keep and do them, that the Lord your God...will love you and bless you and multiply you; He will also bless the fruit of your womb and the fruit of your land...You shall be blessed above all peoples; there shall not be a male or female barren among you...And the Lord will take away from you all sickness, and will afflict you with none of the terrible diseases of Egypt which you have known...."[106]

Do you want your land, which provides your food, to be healed? "If My people who are called by My name will humble themselves, and pray and seek My face, and turn from their wicked ways, then I will hear from heaven, and will forgive their sin and heal their land."[107]

Do you want to be healed? "For the hearts of this people have grown dull. Their ears are hard of hearing, and their eyes they have closed, lest they should see with their eyes and hear with their ears, lest they should understand with their hearts and turn, so that I should heal them."[108]

Do you want health without complying with the conditions? It won't work. "It is through faith in Jesus Christ that the truth is accepted in the heart and the human agent is purified and cleansed. Jesus was 'wounded for our transgressions, he was bruised for our iniquities: the chastisement of our peace was upon him; and with his stripes we are healed.' Is it possible to be healed, while knowingly committing sin?—No; it is genuine faith that says, I know that I have committed sin, but that Jesus has pardoned my sin; and hereafter I will resist temptation in and through His might."[109]

---

[105] Proverbs 4:20-23
[106] Deuteronomy 7:12-15
[107] 2 Chronicles 7:14
[108] Matthew 13:15
[109] White, E. G. (1894) Words to the Young. *The Youth's Instructor.* (February 15, 1894, paragraph 5).

We see, then, that the Lord brings health through His word, through the promises that it contains, through surrender to that word, and through compliance with its conditions. But we also see from this same word that there is an enemy on the loose that we have to watch out for.

CHAPTER NINE

Enemy Warfare

There Is an Enemy

In 1 Peter 5:8 we read, "Be sober, be vigilant; because your adversary the devil walks about like a roaring lion, seeking whom he may devour." There is an enemy who would like nothing more than to destroy us, and thus hurt God, whom he hates. And this controversy between God and the devil can be played out in the life and health of a believer. We see this happening in the life of Job.

In Job chapter 3 and verses 3 through 7 we read, "the Lord said to Satan, 'Have you considered My servant Job, that there is none like him on the earth, a blameless and upright man, one who fears God and shuns evil? And still he holds fast to his integrity, although you incited Me against him, to destroy him without cause.' So Satan answered the Lord and said, 'Skin for skin! Yes, all that a man has he will give for his life. But stretch out Your hand now, and touch his bone and his flesh, and he will surely curse You to Your face!' And the Lord said to Satan, 'Behold, he is in your hand, but spare his life.' So Satan went out from the presence of the Lord, and struck Job with

147

painful boils from the sole of his foot to the crown of his head. And he took for himself a potsherd with which to scrape himself while he sat in the midst of the ashes."

In this story, we find several interesting points that we must consider. First of all, there is a controversy between God and Satan (the word Satan means accuser), where Satan makes accusations to and against God. God could either enter into an argument with Satan (which He never does) and say, "No, you are wrong," while Satan counters with, "No, I am right," and so continue back and forth. But instead, God allows Satan to prove himself wrong by putting the accusation to the test. Thus, God reveals that He is right, and Satan is wrong, and He does so without entering into an argument with Satan.

You see, it is Satan's character to accuse (to bring false accusations against others in an attempt to condemn them), but that is not God's character. We read, "[Jesus] said to them, 'Do not intimidate anyone or accuse falsely.'" [110] "And Jesus said to her, 'Neither do I condemn you; go and sin no more.'" [111] "Do not think that I shall accuse you to the Father." [112] "And the chief priests accused Him of many things, but He answered nothing." [113] "Angels...do not bring a reviling accusation against [sinners] before the Lord." [114] "Yet Michael the archangel, in contending with the devil, when he disputed about the body of Moses, dared not bring against him a reviling accusation." [115]

So, we clearly see that it is not God's character to accuse. And it is not the practice of those in whom God's character reigns. You and I will not accuse others when God lives in our hearts, just like the angels don't accuse us.

---

[110] Luke 3:14
[111] John 8:11
[112] John 5:45
[113] Mark 15:3
[114] 2 Peter 2:11
[115] Jude 1:9

148

Another truth that we learn from the story of Job is that when the Lord allows Satan to put his accusation to the test, God sets limits that Satan cannot cross. In the first trial of Job, in Job chapter 1 and verses 6-22, God said, "Behold, all that he has is in your power; only do not lay a hand on his person."[116] And in the second trial in Job 2:1-10, God says, "Behold, he is in your hand, but spare his life."[117] Satan was permitted to test his accusation, but He was not allowed to go a single bit farther than the Lord permitted. There was a definite line that he could not cross. But in this example, "Job is blameless and upright." Is that true of everyone who is afflicted by Satan?

Sometimes people give themselves over to Satan so that he can control them. And when he does, he can cause physical disease or debilities. "As they went out, behold, they brought to Him a man, mute and demon-possessed. And when the demon was cast out, the mute spoke. And the multitudes marveled, saying, 'It was never seen like this in Israel!'"[118] We see here that Satan can cause someone to be mute.

"Then one was brought to Him who was demon-possessed, blind and mute; and He healed him, so that the blind and mute man both spoke and saw."[119] Not only can Satan cause someone to be mute, but he can cause them to be blind as well.

"...a man came to [Jesus], kneeling down to Him and saying, 'Lord, have mercy on my son, for he is an epileptic and suffers severely; for he often falls into the fire and often into the water...' 'Then Jesus answered and said...Bring him here to Me.' And Jesus rebuked the demon, and it came out of him; and the child was cured from that very hour."[120]

This boy had a "medical" condition called epilepsy (seizure disorder), but obviously Jesus didn't just heal him of epilepsy. He cast

---

[116] Job 1:12
[117] Job 2:6
[118] Matthew 9:32,33
[119] Matthew 12:22
[120] Matthew 17:14-18

a demon out of him, and he was cured. So, the devil can cause epilepsy as well. If the devil is seeking whom he may destroy, why is it that we aren't destroyed? It is only by God's divine intervention—His protection—that we are still alive.

This begs the question, are there ways that I can give Satan permission to work his destructive power in my life? What, if anything, will give him permission to work his destructive power in my life, that he would otherwise have no access or no power to do? Let us consider a few modern stories as we contemplate these questions.

Robert

Jack and Sharon were at their wits' end, and the problem was their 5-year-old son, Robert. Every time he was around other people, he would embarrass them by his foul language and sexually-explicit comments. He had a precocious knowledge of things of a sexual nature, and a propensity to try those things out.

One day, Sharon stepped outside for a couple minutes to do something, and when she came back inside, she found that Robert had undressed himself and Rebecca, their 10-month-old daughter, and was about to accost her. They just couldn't leave him alone for a moment, much less take him to church, for he would embarrass everyone around him.

Then one day a special speaker came to their church and was talking about how Satan can gain access even to Christians and cause problems in the home. So, after the meetings, they consulted with the speaker about their situation with Robert.

After questioning them on a number of points, it was discovered that Sharon was not a Christian when Robert was conceived, and that he was conceived during an orgy. Sharon didn't know who the actual father was. But several months later, when she was pregnant with Robert, she learned about and fell in love with Jesus and was baptized into her church. It was shortly after this that Jack met Sharon, and soon they were married. The speaker asked Sharon about whether she had specifically confessed her sin related to Robert's conception, and if she had asked God to block that access point from the enemy. She had not.

So, the speaker, Jack, and Sharon knelt down then and there, and he led Sharon through a prayer of confession and repentance for that sin, asking the Lord to remove the enemy's access to Robert through Sharon's sin at his conception.

That night, as they returned home, they found an entirely different Robert. He was a normal 5-year-old child, with no precocious knowledge, no foul language, and no embarrassing or dangerous behavior. What was the problem? Sharon's unconfessed sin allowed the enemy to have access to Robert and control his behavior. Once that sin was specifically confessed and repented of, the enemy had no more access to Robert, and he was immediately a normal 5-year-old child.

A

A similar problem existed in our family. I had struggled with an addiction for many years, and was never able to overcome. I still was involved in church, and many would have been shocked to know that I had a secret addiction, but it was always there in the background. Two of our children were conceived while I was still struggling with this problem.

My parents had divorced when I was 14 years old, and as a consequence, I had come to believe that the relationship between a parent and child was stronger than the relationship between a husband and wife. The problem was that I really loved my wife. She was my idol. I didn't want anything to come between us. And now, there was a child, whom we will call A, entering our lives who would have a stronger tie to my wife than I did. Needless to say, I was jealous of this new situation.

After A was born, we didn't bond well. She would always cry and fuss when I held her, and I had a hard time controlling my feelings and responses around her. As she grew, she would scream if I was the one to come into the room when she was crying at night, or if I was the one to change her diaper. We just didn't get along. She always wanted Mommy for everything.

Eventually, my addiction became a real problem, and we finally sought counseling. During the counseling process, the counselors led me through prayer to specifically confess and repent of my involvement in many things (including my addiction) and ask for the Lord to close the doors that I had opened to the enemy through my involvement.

We had been staying at a friend's house about an hour from where the counseling appointments were, and we had left A and her younger sibling with a relative during the counseling appointments. That day, as we returned from the counseling appointment, 3-year-old A came running down the yard to meet us. That was not unusual. But what was unusual was that she ran directly to me with open arms, yelling, "Daddy! Daddy!"

She would never have done this before. She would have run to Mommy. After picking her up, my wife and I looked at each other with a questioning look on our faces. This was so unusual. That evening, after tucking A and her sibling into bed, my wife and I were down stairs. My wife was on the phone updating her mother about the events of the day. A called from upstairs needing to go to the bathroom, and my wife asked me to go get her, since she was on the phone. I dreaded being the one to go, because it always turns into a fight with A screaming that she wants Mommy to take her and not me.

As I peeked around the door and looked into the room, A saw me and said excitedly, "Daddy!" and opened her arms for me to pick her up. She willingly let me carry her downstairs to the bathroom, even walking through the room where Mommy was and not making a fuss. I carried her back upstairs when she was done and put her back in bed, and she said, "I love you, Daddy."

I was absolutely shocked! This was an entirely new child, relating to me in an entirely new way. And ever since that day, our relationship has never been strained like it was those first 3 years. When my sin was specifically confessed and forsaken, when I had asked the Lord to help close the door that the enemy had access to our lives, that avenue was closed, and the enemy could not get to A and cause her to respond like before. And when he no longer had that access, our relationship was restored immediately.

<u>A Friend</u>

I have a friend who has dabbled with the occult, and he has some friends who are still in the occult. He was telling me of one of his friends who has the power of astral projection. Astral projection is a willful out-of-body experience where an individual is aware of and "experiences" things in other locations. For instance, this friend claims the ability to "mentally" go into someone's home and listen to the conversations and see what is going on in that home. This "ability" is only through the power of the devil and his evil angels who are present in the home and aware of what is going on there and can communicate that to the individual as it occurs.

Interestingly, this friend with the power of astral projection stated that she can only get into certain homes. What determines what homes she can "get into" or not "get into?" If there are objects in the home that belong to the devil, then she has permission or power to get into that home and observe what is going on inside.

What do you have in your home that belongs to the devil? And what access does he have to your life and your family as you are in possession of those things?

An Acquaintance

An acquaintance of mine tells the story of when he was speaking at a Christian school in Europe. He was encouraging the students to make a total surrender to the Lord and stop dabbling with the world and the enemy's stuff. He talked with them about getting rid of their Hollywood movies, their worldly music, and separating themselves from everything that separates them from the Lord.

Two of the girls who were roommates were particularly touched by the meetings and decided that they would get rid of everything that they could think of that belonged to the enemy. So, after the meeting that night, they went back to their dorm room and began destroying their CD's and DVD's and other items that they knew separated them from God and gave the enemy access to their lives. The one girl even called her mother (it was about 1 or 2 am where her mother lived) and asked her mother to get rid of all of her CD's and other similar stuff at home. Her mother was happy to comply and went about getting rid of those things that night.

As they were finishing with the "house cleaning," one of the girls recognized that the other girl had a symbol from a popular rock band on her jacket and told the other girl that she should remove that symbol from her jacket, because it was a devilish symbol. So, they proceeded to unstitch the patch and remove it. Once it was removed, the girl who owned the jacket yelled out, "Oh! What happened?!" Her roommate asked her what was wrong. "My pain...my back pain...Is gone! It's gone!" She had suffered for several years with back pain that had debilitated her from time to time but had constantly made her life difficult. But once the last vestige of what belonged to the enemy was removed and destroyed, her pain disappeared!

The Daughter of Abraham

We find a similar story in Scripture. "Now [Jesus] was teaching in one of the synagogues on the Sabbath...there was a woman who had a spirit of infirmity eighteen years, and was bent over and could in no way raise herself up...when Jesus saw her, He called her to Him and said to her, 'Woman, you are loosed from your infirmity.' And He laid His hands on her, and immediately she was made straight...ought not this woman, being a daughter of Abraham, whom Satan has bound—think of it—for eighteen years, be loosed from this bond on the Sabbath?'"[121]

This woman with back problems, bent over and unable to straighten up for 18 years, was bound by Satan. We might look at it today and say that she had severe osteoporosis with compression fractures or scoliosis or kyphosis or something similar. If we had the capacity to do x-rays on her spine before Jesus healed her, we might be able to diagnosis her problem. But what was Jesus' response to her situation? Jesus' testimony was that Satan had bound her.

Does Satan do the same thing today? It would be surprising if he doesn't. So, how does he gain access to us? And what can we do to close the door to his access?

Embassies

When I lived in Trinidad & Tobago (T&T), most days I would drive past the United States Embassy. It was a little piece of home in a foreign land. But I, as a U.S. citizen, was subject to the laws and regulations of T&T as long as I lived in T&T. If I broke their law, I was subject to their penalties accordingly.

Let us imagine that a law is passed in T&T that states that all people living in T&T must renounce their country of origin and become citizens of T&T, and that the penalty for not doing so is life in prison. What could I do? One thing I could do is go to the United

---

[121] Luke 13:10-16

States Embassy. Why go there? Because on the grounds of the U.S. Embassy, the laws and regulations of the United States of America are binding, not the laws of T&T. On those grounds, I would not be in violation of the law, because I would be subject to the laws and regulations of the United States, not T&T.

When a nation gives another nation the right to place an embassy in their territory, what they are doing is giving that piece of land to the other country, where that piece of land becomes a part of the other country and is subject to their rules and regulations, not the rules and regulations of the nation that gave the land.

Satan has an embassy, and that embassy is sin. Wherever sin is found, there the rules and regulations of Satan prevail. Sin in your life and my life gives Satan the permission to work in us his way. If it were not for the restraining grace of God, Satan's way would lead to our immediate destruction. Praise God for His restraining, protecting power in our lives!

Let us look more specifically at ways Satan gains access to us to work our ruin, and therefore what we need to do to shut those doors, so he no longer has that access to us.

Don't wander onto Satan's embassy. That is asking for trouble. "If we venture on Satan's ground, we have no assurance of protection from his power. So far as in us lies, we should close every avenue by which the tempter may find access to us."[122]

Remember, Satan cannot force you. He must be invited. "In no case can Satan obtain dominion over the thoughts, words, and actions, unless we voluntarily open the door and invite him to enter. He will then come in and, by catching away the good seed sown in the heart, make of none effect the truth."[123]

---

[122] White, E. G. (1952) *The Adventist Home*. (p. 402). Hagerstown, MD: Review and Herald Publishing Association.
[123] White, E. G. (1952) *The Adventist Home*. (p. 402). Hagerstown, MD: Review and Herald Publishing Association.

We must remain careful and attentive, or the enemy will gain access to us. "If the workers...become careless and inattentive to their eternal interests...The tempter will find access to them. He will spread nets for their feet, and will lead them in uncertain paths. Those only are safe whose hearts are garrisoned with pure principles."[124]

And Satan can gain access to us at the most innocent places—like at our own tables. "'Satan...can find access through perverted appetite, to debase the soul."[125]

It may not just be the table, but anywhere we yield to intemperance, appetite, and passion can be a place that Satan traps us. "...man, through yielding to Satan's temptations to indulge intemperance, brings the higher faculties in subjection to the...appetites and passions, and...surrenders to the control of Satan. And he gains easy access to those who are in bondage to appetite. Through intemperance, some sacrifice one half, and others two thirds, of their physical, mental, and moral powers, and become playthings for the enemy."[126]

If you have a question about something, just ask yourself the question, "Will this decrease the sensitivity of my conscience or encourage temptation?"

"We must abstain from any practice which will blunt the conscience or encourage temptation. We must open no door that will give Satan access to the mind of one human being formed in the image of God."[127]

One of Satan's favorite means to gain access to our lives is through music. "Satan has no objection to music, if he can make that

---

[124] White, E. G. (1920) *The Colporteur Evangelist*. (p. 44). Mountain View, CA: Pacific Press Publishing Association.
[125] White, E. G. (1953) *Colporteur Ministry*. (p. 133). Mountain View, CA: Pacific Press Publishing Association.
[126] White, E. G. (1971) *Confrontation*. (p. 57). Washington, D.C.: Review and Herald Publishing Association.
[127] White, E. G. (1991) *Counsels for the Church*. (p. 105). Napa, ID: Pacific Press Publishing Association.

a channel through which to gain access to the minds of the youth. Anything will suit his purpose that will divert the mind from God, and engage the time which should be devoted to His service. He works through the means which will exert the strongest influence to hold the largest numbers in a pleasing infatuation, while they are paralyzed by his power."[128]

And Satan sometimes gets access to us in more sinister ways. "Satan is finding access to thousands of minds by presenting himself under the guise of departed friends. The Scriptures declare that "the dead know not anything." Ecclesiastes 9:5. Their thoughts, their love, their hatred, have perished. The dead do not hold communion with the living. But true to his early cunning, Satan employs this device in order to gain control of minds."[129]

Where is safety? It is found while abiding in Christ. "Every Christian must stand on guard continually, watching every avenue of the soul where Satan might find access. He must pray for divine help and at the same time resolutely resist every inclination to sin. By courage, by faith, by persevering toil, he can conquer. But let him remember that to gain the victory Christ must abide in him and he in Christ."[130]

But is being tempted a sin? No! Giving in to temptation is a sin. Even Jesus was tempted. But Satan found no access to Him. Unfortunately, he is more successful with us. "In the wilderness of temptation Christ met the great leading temptations that would assail man. There He encountered, single-handed, the wily, subtle foe, and overcame him. The first great temptation was upon appetite; the second, presumption; the third, love of the world. Satan has overcome his millions by tempting them to the indulgence of

---

[128] White, E. G. (1930) *Messages to Young People.* (p. 295). Hagerstown, MD: Review and Herald Publishing Association.
[129] White, E. G. (1911) *The Acts of the Apostles.* (p. 289). Mountain View, CA: Pacific Press Publishing Association.
[130] White, E. G. (1952) *The Adventist Home.* (p. 403). Hagerstown, MD: Review and Herald Publishing Association.

appetite. Through the gratification of the taste, the nervous system becomes excited and the brain power enfeebled, making it impossible to think calmly or rationally. The mind is unbalanced. Its higher, nobler faculties are perverted to serve animal lust, and the sacred, eternal interests are not regarded. When this object is gained, Satan can come with his two other leading temptations and find ready access. His manifold temptations grow out of these three great leading points."[131]

"Not by one word, not by many words, but by every word that God has spoken, shall man live. We cannot disregard one word, however trifling it may seem to us, and be safe. There is not a commandment of the law that is not for the good and happiness of man, both in this life and in the life to come. In obedience to God's law, man is surrounded as with a hedge and kept from the evil. He who breaks down this divinely erected barrier at one point has destroyed its power to protect him; for he has opened a way by which the enemy can enter to waste and ruin."[132]

And John the Baptist had a similar experience. He did all he could to close the door to the enemy, but that doesn't mean that the enemy didn't tempt him. Again, being tempted is not a sin. Giving in to the temptation is. "John did not feel strong enough to stand the great pressure of temptation he would meet in society. He feared his character would be molded according to the prevailing customs of the Jews, and he chose the wilderness as his school, in which his mind could be properly educated and disciplined from God's great book of nature. In the wilderness, John could the more readily deny himself and bring his appetite under control, and dress in accordance to natural simplicity.

---

[131] White, E. G. (1938). *Counsels on Diet and Foods.* (p. 151). Washington D.C.: Review and Herald Publishing Association.
[132] White, E. G. (1896). *Thoughts from the Mount of Blessing.* (p. 52). Mountain View, CA: Pacific Press Publishing Association.

And there was nothing in the wilderness that would take his mind from meditation and prayer. Satan had access to John, even after he had closed every avenue in his power through which he would enter. But his habits of life were so pure and natural that he could discern the foe, and had strength of spirit and decision of character to resist him."[133]

Let us take a closer look at things that you and me b and our families may have been involved in that may give Satan access to us to work out his ruin in us. First of all, there is frank occult involvement.

Occult Involvement

This includes involvement and experience in or use of things like amulets, association with people in witchcraft, astral projection (out of body experiences), astrology (horoscope), automatic writing, blood pacts, bloody Mary (séance), charms, clairvoyance, consulting a channeler, consulting a medium, consulting a psychic, consulting a Spiritist, crystal balls, demonic tongues, Dungeons and Dragons (and other D&D games), fetishism (object worship), fortune telling, games involving occult power, fantasy role-playing games, occult games involving violence, ghosts, good luck charms, hearing voices in your mind, hypnosis, imaginary playmates, magic eight balls, magic rituals, black or white magic, casting magic spells, martial arts, materialization, mental control of others, mental suggestion, mind control, mind swapping, occult music (glorifies Satan), New Age medicine, occult books/literature, omens, Ouija board, palm reading, Roman Catholic amulets, Satan worship, séances, sexual spirits, speaking in a trance, spirit guides, table lifting or body lifting, Tarot cards, telepathy, transcendental meditation, use of magic healing, using spells or curses, visionary dreams (not from God), visualization, voodoo, water witching/dowsing, witchcraft, and Yoga.

---

[133] White, E. G. (1956) *S.D.A. Bible Commentary, Volume 5.* (p. 1115). Washington D.C.: Review and Herald Publishing Association.

Occult Phenomena

But we also must be aware of occult phenomena, such as demonic nightmares, extra sensory perception (ESP), feeling a presence of evil, having objects disappear, hearing unusual sounds or voices, personality changes, seeing a ghost or large dark image, seeing objects move, and supernatural knowledge or strength.

False Teachings

We can also give room for the Enemy to work in our lives through false teachings, such as Animism, Buddhism, Bahaism, Catholicism, Christian Science, Eckankar, Erhard Seminars Training (EST), Father Divine, Herbert W. Armstrong, Hinduism, Inner Peace Movement, Islam, Jehovah's Witness, Kabbala, Knights Templar, Masons, member of a cult, Mormonism, Native American spirit worship, New Age, New Age Seminar, Pantheism, Rosicrucianism, Roy Masters, Science of the Mind, Scientology, Silva mind control, Theosophy, Unification Church (Moonies), Unitarianism, Unity, Way International, Wicca, and others.

Drug Use

The enemy also gains access to us through the use of mind-altering substances, such as alcohol, amphetamines (uppers), cocaine, Ecstasy, glue sniffing, hashish, heroin, LSD, marijuana, narcotics, barbiturates (downers), PCP, peyote, STP, THC, tobacco, and other street drugs.

Entertainment

And the enemy can also gain access to us through entertainment that he has inspired and which we spend the time to read, listen to, and watch. He can gain access to us through books, cartoons, Disney, entertainment television, Hollywood movies, the internet, magazines, news, novels, pornography, social media, video games, worldly music, even worldly music with Christian words, and YouTube, among others.

Come Out!

So, what does the Word warn us about these things? "Finally, brethren, whatever things are true, whatever things are noble, whatever things are just, whatever things are pure, whatever things are lovely, whatever things are of good report, if there is any virtue and if there is anything praiseworthy—meditate on these things."[134]

"'I will dwell in them and walk among them. I will be their God, and they shall be My people.' Therefore 'Come out from among them and be separate, says the Lord. Do not touch what is unclean, and I will receive you. I will be a Father to you, and you shall be My sons and daughters, says the Lord Almighty.'"[135]

"I beseech you therefore, brethren, by the mercies of God, that you present your bodies a living sacrifice, holy, acceptable to God, which is your reasonable service. And do not be conformed to this world, but be transformed by the renewing of your mind, that you may prove what is that good and acceptable and perfect will of God."[136]

"Do not love the world or the things in the world. If anyone loves the world, the love of the Father is not in him. For all that is in the world—the lust of the flesh, the lust of the eyes, and the pride of life—is not of the Father but is of the world. And the world is passing away, and the lust of it; but he who does the will of God abides forever."[137]

"Satan finds in human hearts some point where he can gain a foothold; some sinful desire is cherished, by means of which his temptations assert their power. But Christ declared of Himself: 'The prince of this world cometh, and hath nothing in Me.' John 14:30.

---

[134] Philippians 4:8
[135] 2 Corinthians 6:16-18
[136] Romans 12:1,2
[137] 1 John 2:15-17

Satan could find nothing in the Son of God that would enable him to gain the victory. He had kept His Father's commandments, and there was no sin in Him that Satan could use to his advantage. This is the condition in which those must be found who shall stand in the time of trouble. It is in this life that we are to separate sin from us, through faith in the atoning blood of Christ. Our precious Savior invites us to join ourselves to him, to unite our weakness to His strength, our ignorance to His wisdom, our unworthiness to His merits."[138]

Let us come to the Lord and confess specifically the things that we have been involved in. Let us ask Him specifically to cut the bonds that the enemy has to us through our family's involvement. And let us come free from sin by the grace of God, trusting in Him to accomplish it in us.

Prayer

If you have personally been involved in occult activity, I would recommend that you pray through the following prayer from the heart, sincerely confessing and forsaking each occult activity you were involved in. "Lord, I confess that I participated in _____. I ask Your forgiveness and I renounce that activity. I ask you, Lord Jesus, to take back ground yielded to the enemy through my participation, and I yield that ground to Your control. I pray that You would break any bondage my involvement will have on my children."

If you have been experiencing occult phenomenon, pray and ask the Lord to reveal to you where the source of that phenomenon is coming from, and then confess and forsake each thing, even confessing what your family may have been involved in. In the blank line, put what occult phenomenon you have been experiencing. "I acknowledge that I have been involved in occult activity or that generations of my family were involved in activities that led to ____ _____. I renounce any activity that my family and I were

[138] White, E. G. (1911) *The Great Controversy* (p. 623). Mountain View, CA: Pacific Press Publishing Association.

involved in that led to the _____ I am experiencing. I ask you, Lord Jesus, to take back the ground given to the enemy through my participation, and I yield that ground to Your control."

If you have been involved in false teaching, confess and forsake each false teaching you have been involved in. "I acknowledge my involvement in the false teaching of _____. I ask Your forgiveness and renounce that false belief. I ask You, Lord Jesus, to take back ground I gave to the enemy, and I yield that ground to Your control."

If you have family members who have been involved in occult activities, false beliefs, or any other generational sin that may be giving the enemy access to your life, pray through each thing, confessing it specifically, listing the person involved in the first line, and what activity or belief they were involved in in the second line. "Lord, I confess that _____ participated in _____. I ask Your forgiveness, and I renounce that activity. I ask You, Lord Jesus, to take back the ground they gave to the enemy through their involvement, and I yield that ground to Your control. I pray that You would break any bondage their involvement will have on my children."

If you have been involved in drug use, pray through each drug of abuse you used, confessing and forsaking each one. "Lord, I confess that I gave ground to the enemy through my use of the drug _____. I ask Your forgiveness and renounce that activity. I ask You, Lord Jesus, to take back ground I gave to the enemy, and I yield that ground to Your control."

And if you have been involved in media consumption, confess each type of media you or your family used and renounce it wholeheartedly. "Lord, I confess that I gave ground to the enemy through my reading / listening to / watching _____. I ask Your forgiveness and renounce that activity. I ask You, Lord Jesus, to take back ground I gave to the enemy, and I yield that ground to Your control."

CHAPTER TEN

A Love that Takes

What Do I Do?

N ow that we see our problem more clearly, the question we must ask ourselves is, "What do I do about it?"

1. Come & Take from God's love

Recognizing that God is the only source, we must come Him and take of His love. Imagine with me that you meet someone that you are interested in, and you are thinking about pursuing a relationship with them. There is only one problem. They are mute (cannot speak). Just because they are mute does not mean that a relationship is impossible. It just changes somewhat how you communicate. You may be able to talk to them, but they will either have to use body language, or write what they are thinking.

In pursuing a relationship with God, in coming to Him as your only source, you can talk to Him like you talk to a friend—in prayer. Tell Him what went right and what went wrong. Tell Him how you feel. Tell Him what you are struggling with and what you would like

Him to help you with. He can handle your feelings. If you are angry, frustrated, depressed, or whatever, He can take it. Don't stop talking with Him just because you don't think He would like what you will say. Just keep talking to Him.

Some people recommend following the PRAY acronym (Praise, Repent, Ask, Yield). Praise and thank Him for the blessings in your life. Look for blessings and ways He is helping you. Repent (be sorry for your sin and turn away from it). Ask Him for help to overcome your difficulties and strength to overcome your weaknesses, and Yield yourself to His control, so that He can lead your life in the way that He knows is best.

In this relationship, God rarely speaks directly to us in an audible voice. But He has left us His love letters (the Bible) that we can read. The Bible has all the answers that we need to all of our problems, situations, and questions. The more you read the Bible, the more you understand about God, and the more you find His answers to your questions. When you are in love, you love reading the love letters of your loved one.

And as you learn more about Him and His love for you, you can spend time contemplating His love. There is a law by which the mind operates. That law is: By beholding we become changed (2 Corinthians 3:18). What we spend our time thinking about, contemplating, watching, listening to, hanging out with, etc. we become like, whether we like it or not. That is just how we operate. So, if you want love, you have to spend time contemplating love. And the only place you will find pure love is God. The greatest revelation of the love of God is found in the sacrifice of Jesus on the cross. I recommend you spend a good amount of time every day reading about and contemplating the love of God as manifested in Jesus' sacrifice from the last supper to His death on the cross. You will be immensely blessed by this!

"I saw how...grace could be obtained. Go to your closet, and there alone plead with God: 'Create in me a clean heart, O God; and renew a right spirit within me.' Be in earnest, be sincere. Fervent prayer availeth much. Jacoblike, wrestle in prayer. Agonize. Jesus, in the garden, sweat great drops of blood; you must make an effort. Do not leave your closet until you feel strong in God; then watch, and just as long as you watch and pray you can keep these evil besetments under, and the grace of God can and will appear in you...Come with zeal, and when you sincerely feel that without the help of God you perish, when you pant after Him as the hart panteth after the water brooks, then will the Lord strengthen you speedily. Then will your peace pass all understanding. If you expect salvation, you must pray. Take time. Be not hurried and careless in your prayers. Beg of God to work in you a thorough reformation, that the fruits of His Spirit may dwell in you, and you shine as lights in the world."[139]

Sources

I want to reiterate something very important at this point. Where do you go to for understanding? When you want to be understood, who can you go to? If you need to be accepted, where do you go? What about for security? With whom do you feel secure? And where do you go to for love?

If you honestly take a survey of your life, how many sources do you have? Spouse, parents, children, friends, colleagues? Let me ask a question we asked previously, can another human being be the source of that which you, as a human being, need? No, they can't, because they need the same things too. So, who is your REAL source of that which you need? It is God.

But in reality, is He your only source, or is He only one of your sources? Isaiah reminds us, "O Lord of hosts, God of Israel, the One who dwells between the cherubim, You are God, You alone, of all

---

[139] White, E. G. (1868). *Testimonies for the Church Volume 1*. Page 158. Mountain View, CA: Pacific Press Publishing Association.

the kingdoms of the earth. You have made heaven and earth."[140]
David reminds us, "For You are great, and do wondrous things; You
alone are God."[141]

Paul reminds us, "For by Him all things were created that are in
heaven and that are on earth, visible and invisible, whether thrones or
dominions or principalities or powers. All things were created
through Him and for Him. And He is before all things, and in Him
all things consist."[142]

Your mother is not your source. Your spouse is not your source.
Your child is not your source. Your friend is not your source. Your
dog is not your source. Your cat is not your source. None of these are
your sources. You have only ONE source, and that source is God.

Do you need to belong somewhere and with someone? Go to
God, not to your mother. Do you need to be accepted by someone?
Go to God, not your friend. Do you need to feel secure? Go to God,
not your financial advisor. Do you need harmony? Seek it from God,
not from your spouse.

I picture God above me and everyone else beside me. Vertically,
God is to be my source for everything I need, so what is the purpose
for having horizontal relationships (relationships with other people)?
Others are not there to be my source. Only God is there to be my
source. Others are there to give me an opportunity to give away that
which I took from God. Others are not there for me to take from.
They are there for me to give to.

But, in order to be able to give, I must have something to give.
So how do I get that which I need from God? Besides what I
mentioned previously; I have found that it primarily comes from
trusting in His promises.

Do you need acceptance? God promises you, "But as many as
received Him, to them He gave the right to become children of God,

[140] Isaiah 37:16
[141] Psalm 86:10
[142] Colossians 1:15-17

to those who believe in His name."[143] "But in every nation whoever fears Him and works righteousness is accepted by Him."[144] "Blessed be the God and Father of our Lord Jesus Christ, who has blessed us with every spiritual blessing in the heavenly places in Christ, just as He chose us in Him before the foundation of the world, that we should be holy and without blame before Him in love, having predestined us to adoption as sons by Jesus Christ to Himself, according to the good pleasure of His will, to the praise of the glory of His grace, by which He made us accepted in the Beloved."[145] "For God so loved the world that He gave His only begotten Son, that whoever believes in Him should not perish but have everlasting life. For God did not send His Son into the world to condemn the world, but that the world through Him might be saved."[146]

Do you need belonging? God promises you, "But now, thus says the Lord, who created you, O Jacob, and He who formed you, O Israel: 'Fear not, for I have redeemed you; I have called you by your name; you are Mine.'"[147] "Can a woman forget her nursing child, and not have compassion on the son of her womb? Surely they may forget, yet I will not forget you. See, I have inscribed you on the palms of My hands; your walls are continually before Me."[148] "But when the fullness of the time had come, God sent forth His Son, born of a woman, born under the law, to redeem those who were under the law, that we might receive the adoption as sons. And because you are sons, God has sent forth the Spirit of His Son into your hearts, crying out, "Abba, Father!" Therefore you are no longer a slave but a son, and if a son, then an heir of God through Christ."[149] "Behold what manner of love the Father has bestowed on us, that we

---

[143] John 1:12
[144] Acts 10:35
[145] Ephesians 1:3-6
[146] John 3:16,17
[147] Isaiah 43:1
[148] Isaiah 49:15-16
[149] Galatians 4:4-7

should be called children of God! Therefore the world does not know us, because it did not know Him."[150]

Do you need security? God promises you, "The angel of the Lord encamps all around those who fear Him, and delivers them."[151] "And my God shall supply all your need according to His riches in glory by Christ Jesus."[152] "Fear not, for I am with you; be not dismayed, for I am your God. I will strengthen you, Yes, I will help you, I will uphold you with My righteous right hand.'"[153] "When you pass through the waters, I will be with you; and through the rivers, they shall not overflow you. When you walk through the fire, you shall not be burned, nor shall the flame scorch you."[154] "No weapon formed against you shall prosper, and every tongue which rises against you in judgment you shall condemn. This is the heritage of the servants of the Lord, and their righteousness is from Me,' says the Lord."[155]

Do you need understanding? God promises you, "Surely He has borne our griefs and carried our sorrows; yet we esteemed Him stricken, smitten by God, and afflicted."[156] "For we do not have a High Priest who cannot sympathize with our weaknesses, but was in all points tempted as we are, yet without sin. Let us therefore come boldly to the throne of grace, that we may obtain mercy and find grace to help in time of need."[157]

Do you need truth? God promises you, "The entirety of Your word is truth, and every one of Your righteous judgments endures forever."[158] "Sanctify them by Your truth. Your word is truth."[159] "Jesus said to him, 'I am the way, the truth, and the life. No one comes to

---

[150] 1 John 3:1
[151] Psalm 34:7
[152] Philippians 4:19
[153] Isaiah 41:10
[154] Isaiah 43:2
[155] Isaiah 54:17
[156] Isaiah 53:4
[157] Hebrews 4:15,16
[158] Psalm 119:160
[159] John 17:17

the Father except through Me.'"[160] "Then Jesus said to those Jews who believed Him, 'If you abide in My word, you are My disciples indeed. And you shall know the truth, and the truth shall make you free.'"[161]

Do you need forgiveness? God promises you, "He has not dealt with us according to our sins, nor punished us according to our iniquities. For as the heavens are high above the earth, so great is His mercy toward those who fear Him; as far as the east is from the west, so far has He removed our transgressions from us."[162] "Who is a God like You, pardoning iniquity and passing over the transgression of the remnant of His heritage? He does not retain His anger forever, because He delights in mercy. He will again have compassion on us, and will subdue our iniquities. You will cast all our sins into the depths of the sea."[163] "If we confess our sins, He is faithful and just to forgive us our sins and to cleanse us from all unrighteousness."[164]

Do you need joy? God promises you, "You will show me the path of life; In Your presence is fullness of joy; at Your right hand are pleasures forevermore."[165] "Restore to me the joy of Your salvation, and uphold me by Your generous Spirit."[166] "For God gives wisdom and knowledge and joy to a man who is good in His sight; but to the sinner He gives the work of gathering and collecting, that he may give to him who is good before God. This also is vanity and grasping for the wind."[167] "Your words were found, and I ate them, and Your word was to me the joy and rejoicing of my heart; for I am called by Your name, O Lord God of hosts."[168] "'These things I have spoken to you, that My joy may remain in you, and that your joy may be full."[169] "Until now you have asked nothing in My name. Ask, and you will

---

[160] John 14:6
[161] John 8:31,32
[162] Psalm 103:10-12
[163] Micah 7:18,19
[164] 1 John 1:9
[165] Psalm 16:11
[166] Psalm 51:12
[167] Ecclesiastes 2:26
[168] Jeremiah 15:16
[169] John 15:11

receive, that your joy may be full."[170] "But now I come to You, and these things I speak in the world, that they may have My joy fulfilled in themselves."[171]

Do you need peace? God promises you, "The Lord will give strength to His people; the Lord will bless His people with peace."[172] "You will keep him in perfect peace, whose mind is stayed on You, because he trusts in You."[173] "I will hear what God the Lord will speak, for He will speak peace to His people and to His saints; but let them not turn back to folly."[174] "Peace I leave with you, My peace I give to you; not as the world gives do I give to you. Let not your heart be troubled, neither let it be afraid."[175] "These things I have spoken to you, that in Me you may have peace. In the world you will have tribulation; but be of good cheer, I have overcome the world.'"[176] "Now may the God of hope fill you with all joy and peace in believing, that you may abound in hope by the power of the Holy Spirit."[177]

Do you need compassion? God promises you, "But You, O Lord, are a God full of compassion, and gracious, longsuffering and abundant in mercy and truth."[178] "But when He saw the multitudes, He was moved with compassion for them, because they were weary and scattered, like sheep having no shepherd."[179]

Do you need hope? God promises you, "Be of good courage, and He shall strengthen your heart, all you who hope in the Lord."[180] "It is good that one should hope and wait quietly for the salvation of the Lord."[181] "For I know the thoughts that I think toward you, says the Lord, thoughts of peace and not of evil, to give you a future and a

---

[170] John 16:24
[171] John 17:13
[172] Psalm 29:11
[173] Isaiah 26:3
[174] Psalm 85:8
[175] John 14:27
[176] John 16:33
[177] John 15:13
[178] Psalm 86:15
[179] Matthew 9:36
[180] Psalm 31:24
[181] Lamentations 3:26

hope."[182] "Let not your heart be troubled; you believe in God, believe also in Me. In My Father's house are many mansions; if it were not so, I would have told you. I go to prepare a place for you. And if I go and prepare a place for you, I will come again and receive you to Myself; that where I am, there you may be also."[183] "Now may the God of hope fill you with all joy and peace in believing, that you may abound in hope by the power of the Holy Spirit."[184]

"When the promises of God are freely and fully accepted, heaven's brightness is brought into the life."[185] You and I primarily take of God's love by becoming familiar with His promises, reciting them, using them in times of need, allowing them to be the theme of our thoughts, and believing them.

2. Accept A New Heart / New Love

In addition to praying, reading His Word, and contemplating His love, we must accept the new heart God desires to give us, which operates by the Law of Life—take to give.

I don't know if you have seen a heart transplant surgery before, or if you have been involved in one or had a friend or family member that did. But if you have, there is one thing you will quickly realize, and that is that a heart transplant is not painless! Why would someone go through a heart transplant? Why would you participate in a heart transplant, and what are the steps you need to consider as you consider accepting that new heart?

1. You must have an incurable, fatal heart condition.

If your heart can be cured or managed any other way, you are not a candidate for a heart transplant. It is only those who have an

---

[182] Jeremiah 29:11
[183] John 14:1-3
[184] Romans 15:3
[185] White, E. G. (1933) *A Call to Medical Evangelism and Health Education*. (P 26). Nashville, TN: Southern Publishing Association.

incurable heart condition that is fatal who are eligible for a heart transplant.

2. *You must trust the Surgeon and give consent.*

The Surgeon, Christ, will not take you to surgery without your consent. He respects your freedom of choice and will not force you to do good or to do wickedness. So, you must give Him consent to perform the procedure before He will perform it. But if you are going to give Him consent, you must trust Him.

Imagine that you are in need of a heart transplant, and you are at the hospital, all hooked up and ready for surgery, and the surgeon walks in, and he's a young guy with barely three hairs growing on his upper lip. You ask him how many of these procedures he has done before, and he somewhat sheepishly tells you that this will be his first time. Are you going to let him cut you open? I wouldn't! I would be looking for a second opinion. I want a surgeon who has done the procedure many times before and has a very good success record.

Jesus has performed this procedure millions of times and has never lost a case. You can trust Him with your heart transplant.

3. *You must be willing to go through the pain.*

As mentioned before, open heart surgery is not painless. To begin with, a scalpel is used to cut the skin from the center of the lower neck to just below the breast bone. Then a saw is used to cut the breast bone in two from top to bottom. Next, rib spreaders are placed in the chasm and cranked by hand to spread the chest apart so the surgeon can see inside. Next, the left lung is pushed aside gently, and the sack containing the heart is cut so the heart can be delivered. Finally, the surgeon holds the heart in his hand and can begin working on the heart.

At the end of the surgery, everything happens in reverse. But the breast bone is still not attached, so the surgeon takes a large, curved needle with a wire attached to it and pushes it through the breast bone on one side and then on the other. He draws the wire through and then uses pliers to "twisty-tie" the two sides of the breast bone together. He does that several times down the breast bone. And, finally, the skin is stapled together.

The patient may have been asleep during the surgery, but after the surgery they have to wake up. And when they wake up, it hurts! Their back hurts. Their chest hurts. Their throat hurts. Praise God for something to dull the pain!

But, in order to not develop pneumonia, the patient is then instructed to breathe deeply and is given a device that helps them to practice breathing deeply. Why do they need to be encouraged to breathe deeply? It is because the wire twisty-ties do not hold the breast bone together perfectly, and every time the patient breathes deeply, coughs, sneezes, or laughs, the one side of the breast bone rubs against the other side, and there is intense pain. For the sake of any friends that you visit in the hospital after open heart surgery (or any surgery for that matter), please don't make them laugh!

If you are going to receive a new heart, you have to be willing to face the pain. In receiving this new heart, there is pain as well. There is confession. There is repentance. There is humiliation. There is giving up one's idols and dreams. There is letting go of one's possessions. There is a complete surrender of one's self to the Surgeon.

4. There must be a donor with a good heart.

If you have an incurable, fatal heart condition, and the donor has another incurable, fatal heart condition, there is no point in having the surgery. If you are going to undergo the surgery, you must have a donor that has a good heart to exchange for your bad one.

God knew this, and after looking all over and finding no suitable heart, He decided that His heart was the only one that would work.

5. The donor must die.

Of course, we know that if you are going to receive a new heart, the former owner of that heart must die. Jesus knew that too, and when He decided that only His heart would suffice, He knew that He must die in the process. But He loved us so much that He was willing to make the sacrifice for us.

6. The recipient must die...and be revived.

Many people don't realize that the recipient of the new heart must die as well. You see, the surgeon has to cut out the old heart before putting the new one in place.

I have been in open heart surgery, and it can be quite nerve-racking. The bypass machine has been pumping blood through the body but not through the heart for quite some time. When the new heart is finally sutured together, blood is allowed to flow through the heart as the bypass machine ports are removed. But the heart isn't beating.

The surgeon takes small metal paddles and places them in the chest next to the heart and gives the heart a shock. Then there is nervous waiting. No heartbeat. The surgeon shocks again. More nervous waiting. Still no heartbeat. He reaches into the chest and rhythmically squeezes the heart in his hand for a while, circulating blood to the body and especially the brain. He then shocks the heart a third time and waits. Still no heartbeat. You can feel the tension in the room. If this heart doesn't beat, all will be for nothing. One more shock, and the heart responds with a disorganized quivering for a few seconds. And then a sigh of relief spreads throughout the operating room as the heart begins to beat in a regular fashion. The dead has been revived!

7. You must follow the Surgeon's instructions for the rest of your life.

Now that you have successfully survived the heart transplant, you must follow the Surgeon's instructions, for you are no longer in possession of your heart. You are in possession of His. And His heart must be treated a certain way in order for it to be preserved. If you treat that new heart like you treated the old one, the same terminal condition will result. No, you must follow His instructions and do so for the rest of your life.

But how do you obtain this new heart? What is the missing ingredient? It is faith. The new heart is a gift of God's grace, received and accepted by faith. But let us look at this a little closer so that we understand what faith is and how it is exercised. For this, we will go back to the very beginning.

<u>Creation & Faith</u>

"Then God said, 'Let there be light'; and there was light."[186] "Then God said, 'Let there be a firmament in the midst of the waters, and let it divide the waters from the waters.' Thus God made the firmament, and divided the waters which were under the firmament from the waters which were above the firmament; and it was so."[187] "Then God said, 'Let the waters under the heavens be gathered together into one place, and let the dry land appear'; and it was so."[188] "Then God said, 'Let the earth bring forth grass, the herb that yields seed, and the fruit tree that yields fruit according to its kind, whose seed is in itself, on the earth'; and it was so."[189] "Then God said, 'Let there be lights in the firmament of the heavens to divide the day from the night; and let them be for signs and seasons, and for days and years; and let them be for lights in the firmament of the heavens to

---

[186] Genesis 1:3
[187] Genesis 1:6,7
[188] Genesis 1:9
[189] Genesis 1:11

give light on the earth'; and it was so."[190] "Then God said, 'Let the waters abound with an abundance of living creatures, and let birds fly above the earth across the face of the firmament of the heavens.' So God created great sea creatures and every living thing that moves, with which the waters abounded, according to their kind, and every winged bird according to its kind. And God saw that it was good."[191] "Then God said, 'Let the earth bring forth the living creature according to its kind: cattle and creeping thing and beast of the earth, each according to its kind'; and it was so."[192]

Here we see that God spoke everything into existence by the power of His word. He spoke and it was. It wasn't that He spoke the thing, and then had to accomplish what He spoke. His word is creative and accomplishes the thing that is spoken. God's word can create something from nothing: light, atmosphere, land, stars and planets, plants, and animals. All were created by the power that is in God's spoken word.

Not only is His word creative, but His word is recreative. In the book of John, we find that, "In the beginning was the Word, and the Word was with God, and the Word was God. He was in the beginning with God. All things were made through Him, and without Him nothing was made that was made. In Him was life, and the life was the light of men...And the Word became flesh and dwelt among us, and we beheld His glory, the glory as of the only begotten of the Father, full of grace and truth."[193] So, we see that Jesus was the one who spoke all things into existence. He was the creator of all the universe and created it all by the power of His word. But John helps us to realize that not only did He speak and create, but that He *was* the Word, and that the God who was the Word, who spoke all things

---

[190] Genesis 1:14,15
[191] Genesis 1:20,21
[192] Genesis 1:24
[193] John 1:1-4,14

into being from nothing, that same Word became a human being and lived among us.

In the life and ministry of Jesus, we see His recreative power at work. In Matthew 9 and verses 27 through 30 we read, "When Jesus departed from there, two blind men followed Him, crying out and saying, 'Son of David, have mercy on us!' And when He had come into the house, the blind men came to Him. And Jesus said to them, 'Do you believe that I am able to do this?' They said to Him, 'Yes, Lord.' Then He touched their eyes, saying, 'According to your faith let it be to you.' And their eyes were opened."

This was only one representative healing among thousands of people whom Jesus healed. But in healing people, there is an additional factor that we must consider. In creation, Adam and Eve could give no consent in their own creation. But with recreation, with healing, each person that Jesus healed exercised faith in Him and His ability to heal them.

God allows for complete freedom of choice. He is not interested in robots serving Him. He wants creatures who can choose to serve, creatures who can love. In giving us the capacity to choose and to love, God respects our choice, even when it is not a good one. Jesus would not heal someone who had no faith in Him, because to do otherwise would be to force good (healing) on that person, and God will not force good on you just as he will not force evil on you. You must choose. Therefore, healing is a consensual act between God who has the power to heal, and a creature who consents to the healing.

Let us take one more example when considering faith and what it is. Matthew 8 and verses 5 through 13 reveals, "Now when Jesus had entered Capernaum, a centurion came to Him, pleading with Him, saying, 'Lord, my servant is lying at home paralyzed, dreadfully tormented.' And Jesus said to him, 'I will come and heal him.' The centurion answered and said, 'Lord, I am not worthy that You should come under my roof. But only speak a word, and my servant will be healed. For I also am a man under authority, having soldiers under me. And I say to this one, 'Go,' and he goes; and to another, 'Come,' and he comes; and to my servant, 'Do this,' and he does it.' When Jesus heard it, He marveled, and said to those who followed, 'Assuredly, I say to you, I have not found such great faith, not even in Israel...' Then Jesus said to the centurion, 'Go your way; and as you have believed, so let it be done for you.' And his servant was healed that same hour."

If Jesus says that something is faith and is great faith, should we not pay attention? Jesus said that the centurion had faith, great faith. So, what was that faith? The centurion came to Jesus, expecting that Jesus had the power to heal his servant. When Jesus said that He would go and heal the servant, the centurion showed that he believed Jesus did not need to go to the home to heal. He believed that Jesus was God and had creative power in His word. All He needed to do was speak the word and his servant would be healed. That is faith. It is knowing that the word of God has power in itself, expecting the word of God itself to do what it says, and depending upon the word itself to accomplish it.

How much righteousness resides in your heart? None. Then, just as in creation, God must speak righteousness into existence in your heart from nothing.

"'He spake, and it was.' Before He spoke, there were no worlds; after He spoke, the worlds were there. The word of God spoken by Jesus Christ is able to cause that to exist which has no existence before the word is spoken, and which, except for that word, never could have existence. In the same way precisely it is in man's life. In man's life there is no righteousness. In man there is no righteousness from which righteousness can appear in his life. But God has set forth Christ to declare righteousness unto and upon man. Christ has spoken the word only, and in the darkened void of man's life there is righteousness to everyone who will receive it. Where, before the word is received, there was neither righteousness nor anything which could possibly produce righteousness, after the word is received, there is perfect righteousness and the very Fountain from which it springs. The word of God received by faith—that is, the word of God expected to do what that word says and depended upon to do what it says—produces righteousness in the man and in the life where there never was any before; precisely as, in the original creation, the word of God produces worlds where there never were any worlds before. He has spoken, and it is so to everyone that believeth: that is, to everyone that receiveth. The word itself produces it."[194]

So, how do you obtain the new heart that you desperately need but which you cannot produce? It is in the same way. God has given His word, "I will give you a new heart and put a new spirit within you; I will take the heart of stone out of your flesh and give you a heart of flesh." Ezekiel 36:26. The creative word has spoken it, but in redemption, there must be the consent of the recipient. You must go to the restaurant and take what you need. You must agree to undergo the heart transplant operation, allowing the Surgeon to do His work. When faith takes ahold of the creative word, that which the creative word has spoken is so, and will be realized in your life at the very time when it is needed most. You hope for the promise which you do not see in reality. But "faith is the substance of things hoped for, the evidence of things not seen."[195] That means that faith, by the power of the word, allows that which is not in existence to become reality. And faith itself is the evidence of that which you cannot see yet.

Faith and trust are inseparable, so can you have faith in someone and distrust them at the same time? No, you cannot. So, faith in God's word means that you trust that word, and it means you trust the one who spoke that word.

---

[194] Jones, A.T., Waggoner, E.J. (1995) *Lessons on Faith: A Selection of Articles & Sermons.* (p. 13) Brushton, N.Y.: Teach Services.
[195] Hebrews 11:1

CHAPTER ELEVEN

A Love that Values

3. Accept the Divine Exchange at the Cross

B y faith, become a participant in the divine exchange at the cross, where you receive Jesus' past as your own, and He takes from you your past. You cease to be the victim and the perpetrator and you go free! But be careful to not pick up your burden again. It is so easy for us to come to Jesus with our burdens in prayer and mention them to Him but not leave them at the cross. We walk away still carrying our burden.

For instance, suppose there is a parent who is concerned about their child. Perhaps the child is pursuing a life of self-destruction through substances, addictions, and other harmful lifestyle behaviors. The parent, if they are a praying parent, will most likely bring that child to God in prayer daily or multiple times through the day. They will ask for the Lord to protect and convert their child and generally intervene in their life in order to save them.

But then what does the parent do? They go throughout their day worrying about their child and what they are doing and whether they will ever respond to God again. That is not bringing your burden to the cross and leaving it there. That is bringing the burden to the cross and then taking it with you and bearing it yourself.

Does God love your child? Of course, He does. How much does He love your child? More than you do or less than you do? More than you do. How much more than you do? Infinitely more than you do. Does God have power? Yes, He has power. Does He have more power than you do? Of course, He does. How much more power does God have than you? Infinitely more power. So, if it is for the good, and if it does not violate the child's rights, will God use His infinite power to work out salvation for the child whom He loves infinitely? Yes, He will!

The next question is not an easy one in reality. Can you trust God to work out the salvation of your child that you prayed for? "Of course," you say. But can you, in reality? If you can trust God and if you do trust God to work it out, then you have nothing to worry about.

"Faith is the substance of things hoped for, the evidence of things not seen." Hebrews 11:1. So faith takes hold of the love of God and believes that He will work out what is best in His own time and way, and believes it to such a degree that the thing to come is in my mind currently a reality—so real that it is like physical substance in front of me and evidence that can be used in a court of law. And if there is a present reality of what is to come, I have nothing to worry about, because it is already taken care of in Christ.

So, when you bring your burdens to the Lord, by faith leave them there. Let the Lord work it out in His own time and way and just trust that He will work it out infinitely better than you ever could. His death on the cross proves His love for you and for those you love. His love is infinite, and you can trust such an infinite love.

Valuable

What makes something worth what it is worth? Is it what it is made of? Is it based upon what it can do? Ultimately, value is determined by what someone (the highest bidder) is willing to pay for the thing. So, how much are you worth? Before we answer that question, let us take a detour for a little while.

The earth that you and I live on is a beautiful place. And it is relatively large. The Earth's circumference is 24,901 miles, which means that if you were to drive around the world in a straight line at the equator at 70 mph, it would take you 355.7 hours, or almost 15 days straight to drive around the world once.

And the earth has a mass of 5,973,600,000,000,000,000,000,000 kg. If you were to be able to bench press 200 pounds, and you could do so every second, you would have to bench press at that rate for 1,960,000,000,000,000,000,000 years to eventually lift the same weight as the world is.

If you have a fast car, you can drive over 200 mph, but the earth rotates at about 1,000 mph, and its orbital speed is 66,611mph. That's fast! If you drive in the right direction at the right spot on the earth, you can be going 67,811 mph!

And, of course, the earth is only one of eight or nine planets in our solar system. Mercury, Venus, Earth, Mars, Jupiter, Saturn, Uranus, Neptune, (and maybe Pluto?). And all of these planets are orbiting around the sun. Our sun is a medium-sized star that is 93 million miles away from us. Even at the immense speeds of light, it takes over 8 seconds for light to travel from the sun to earth. At its surface, the sun is 10,000 degrees Fahrenheit. The sun is so big that if the earth were the size of a golf ball, the sun would have a diameter of 15 feet. You could fit 960,000 earths inside the sun. That is enough golf balls to fill a school bus.

And when we compare the earth to other planets, we find that it is slightly larger than 3 or 4 of the other planets. But it is much smaller than the rest. But when we compare our planets to stars, there is very little comparison.

Betelgeuse is called the "orange giant," and is a part of the Orion constellation. It is 427 light years away from us and is twice the size of the Earth's orbit around the sun. If the Earth were the size of a golf ball, Betelgeuse would be the size of 6 Empire State Buildings on top of each other! That is 612 stories tall. You could fit 262,000,000,000,000 earths inside of Betelgeuse. That is enough golf balls to fill the Superdome in Louisiana 3,000 times!

Mu Cephei is 3,000 light years away from us. If the Earth were the size of a golf ball, Mu Cephi would be the size of 2 Golden Gate Bridges end to end! That is a 2.4-mile diameter! You could fit 2,700,000,000,000,000 (quadrillion) earths inside of Mu Cephi.

To get an idea of how large a number quadrillion is, consider that 1 million seconds ago was 11.5 days ago, 1 billion seconds ago was 31.7 years ago, 1 trillion seconds ago was 31,688 years ago, and 1 quadrillion seconds ago was 31,688,088 years ago. A quadrillion is a ridiculously large number. And you could fit 2.7 quadrillion earths inside of Mu Cephi.

But the largest star that we know of is called VY Canis Majoris (the Big Dog). If the Earth were the size of a golf ball, Canis Majoris would be the size of Mt. Everest, 5.5 miles from sea level to the peak. You could fit 7 quadrillion earths inside of Canis Majoris. That is enough golf balls to cover the entire surface of Alabama with golf balls 3.6 feet deep!

When we look into the sky on a dark night, many times we think we are seeing stars. But if we only looked at those "stars" with more and more powerful telescopes, we would notice that some of them are not stars. They are galaxies. These galaxies are made up of many stars, with anywhere from 10,000,000 to 100,000,000,000,000 stars in a single galaxy. And if we had more and more powerful telescopes, we would probably find much more than we now know.

The average distance between stars in our galaxy is 4.3 light years. That is equal to 5,878,625,000,000 miles. These stars that are close to us make up the Milky Way Galaxy, which is our galaxy. The Milky Way Galaxy contains approximately 300,000,000,000 (billion) stars, and it is about 10,000 light years thick (or 58,786,250,000,000,000 miles), and about 100,000 light years wide (or 587,862,500,000,000,000 miles).

The largest galaxy that we know of is inside the Abell 2029 cluster. It contains approximately 100,000,000,000,000 stars. The most distant known galaxy, UDFj-39546284, is approximately 13.37 billion light years from Earth. That is equivalent to 78,597,216,250,000,000,000 miles away from earth. It is estimated that the entire "known universe" is 91 billion light years across. That is 546,700,000,000,000,000,000,000 miles!

There are an estimated 200 billion galaxies and 1,000,000,000,000,000,000,000,000 (septillion) stars in the entire observable universe.

To get an idea of what 1 septillion is like, imagine that you go down to the beach, and you take a pair of tweezers and a bag with you. You start picking up grains of sand one by one until you have picked up the entire beach and ocean floor and land mass near you, and then you work your way around all of the beaches and islands and continents around the entire world. Once you have finished picking up every single piece of sand on planet earth, you will have approximately 1 septillion pieces of sand. This is how many stars that are estimated to be in the observable universe.

And God promised Abraham, "blessing I will bless you, and multiplying I will multiply your descendants as the stars of the heaven and as the sand which is on the seashore; and your descendants shall possess the gate of their enemies."[196]

On August 6, 1945, the United States dropped a nuclear bomb on the Japanese city of Hiroshima. That nuclear bomb released an estimated 6.0×10^{13} Joules of energy. But such a devastating

---

[196] Genesis 22:17

explosion is nothing compared to the sun. The sun releases 3.8 X 10^{26} Joules of energy in 1 second. That is 6,333,333,333,333 (trillion) times the Hiroshima nuclear bomb every second!

That is incredible power! But our sun is not the most powerful thing out there. When it comes to the release of power, the most powerful things in the universe that we know of are quasars. A quasar can release 1.95 X 10^{39} Joules of energy in 1 second. That is 5,100,000,000,000 (trillion) times the power of the sun every second! And where do the stars and quasars get their power?

"By the word of the Lord the heavens were made, and all the host of them by the breath of His mouth."[197] God is the power behind these universal powerhouses.

And is God bigger or smaller than the creation that He has made? Can He create into a space where He is not at or has no access to? No, of course not. So, He is bigger than His creation.

Imagine with me about heaven. What would it be like to be there? Imagine the city of God, made from 12 different jewels, and its 12 gates, each made from a single pearl. Imagine streets that are pure gold, so pure that they are transparent. Imagine the river of life that contains living, pure, clean water miles wide. And imagine the tree of life, with one trunk on one side of the river of life and one trunk on the other side coming together in the middle—a tree miles high and miles wide! Imagine the angel choirs of millions of voices blending in perfect harmony and perfect timing, singing praises to the God who created all of this beauty. Just imagine what it would be like to be there. If you went there, would you ever want to leave?

Now, imagine God as the center of all worship and adoration. Imagine that beings are constantly singing praises to Him and blessing Him for His holiness and love. Imagine Him surrounded by such beauty that we can't describe. Imagine that He is bigger than all of the

---

[197] Psalm 33:6

universe and so powerful that everything comes into existence just because He speaks it.

And now, imagine two small creatures on a small planet in the vast shores of the universe rebel against God and choose their own way rather than His perfect way. It would be like two microscopic viruses on the surface of a single grain of sand down at the beach. How easy would it have been for God to just blot out their existence?

But no, God had a greater plan. Instead of blotting out those two specks and their planet (so insignificant in the expanse of the universe), God decided that He was going to become one of them in an attempt to rescue and redeem them from their rebellion and restore them to friendship with Himself.

An angel was sent to Mary, and when she consented to be a part of God's plan to become man, God packaged Himself in a single cell in Mary's womb. God, who is greater than the universe we have been talking about, became the smallest, most insignificant and vulnerable form of life possible—a single cell.

That cell divided from one into two, then two into four, then four into eight cells. It became a morula and then a blastula and started to form ectoderm, mesoderm, and endoderm. It started to form a vertebral column and a head, and then budded legs and arms and eventually feet and hands. Its heart began to beat and its bones began to form. It twitched and moved and sucked its thumb, all inside of Mary's womb.

Then one day, it happened. After a bumpy ride on a donkey from Nazareth to Bethlehem, Mary's water broke, and it was time for Jesus to be delivered into the world. But it was a cold, dismal, uncaring world that He was delivered into. With only stinky shepherds and animals to welcome the birth of God who became man, Jesus' only place to sleep was an animal's feeding trough.

Poor as they were, it was not likely an easy existence for Joseph and Mary in Bethlehem. Joseph had to work hard and long to try to support the family and find a place for them to stay, for the stable could only be lived in for a short time.

None of the religious leaders came to see and worship the God-man who had come into the world. Everyone around only saw a typical baby. No one, even Jesus' parents, really understood the significance of Who He really was.

By the age of two, His life was threatened, and His family had to flee for their lives, exiles in a foreign land. And when they returned home, there was no greeting party to meet them and escort them to the palace in Jerusalem. So, they lived a life of common laborers in Nazareth. Unrecognized and unappreciated.

Jesus' life was lived to bless and lift up others. Everything He did was for the sake of helping others. He thought of them, prayed for them, treated them as they should be treated, and sacrificed Himself for their good. But all the time, He was misunderstood and treated with suspicion and even hatred.

The religious leaders were constantly sending spies to catch Him in His words so that they could condemn Him to death. Several times, His Father had to miraculously preserve His life, because the people hated Him for what He said and tried to stone Him or throw Him off of a cliff.

Was He discouraged by this? Did He stop His work and go back to heaven to leave us to our stubborn, sin-filled, rebellious lives? No! "For God so loved the world that He gave His only begotten Son, that whoever believes in Him should not perish but have everlasting life."[198]

Man's rebellion earned for him the penalty of death, and Jesus must come to pay that penalty for man, the innocent for the guilty. Jesus' perfect life earned for Him the reward of eternal life, and He came to give that reward to man. Jesus could not succeed in His mission to rescue us if He sinned—even once. Nor could He succeed

[198] John 3:16

in His mission if He did not die the death we deserve. The mission must be complete.

Rejected and despised by those He came to save, He had only thoughts of good for them and acted only for their restoration. But men misinterpreted His works and motives, and they would not allow themselves to be convicted by His perfect life that their lives were sinful and deserving of death. He came as the light of the world, but they loved the darkness and would not come to the light.

So, in the dark of night, they came and arrested Him. During the night, they arraigned Him before the highest council of their nation. They condemned Him before the Romans. They called for His death, saying, "His blood be on us and on our children."[199] With a cat o' nine tails, he was whipped 78 times, turning His back and sides into a bruised and bloody mess. Thorns were twisted into a make-shift crown and then pounded into his head with the blows of a staff.

He was mocked, spat upon, punched and kicked. Pieces of His beard were ripped out, and eventually, those hands which had been so busy helping others were nailed to the cross. Those feet which had walked so far to reach others with messages of love and restoration, were spiked to that tree. The One who had only love was shown only hatred. The One who sought to restore was the object of destruction.

But far beyond the physical pain and torture that He endured, the torture of Jesus' soul was the hiding of His Father's face. As Jesus took the sins of the whole world upon Himself—as He became sin for us—those sins separated Him, who had always been one with the Father, from His Father. He became the object of His Father's wrath against sin and suffered the second death for each of us.

Why? Why go through the torture? Why suffer so much? Why pay such a tremendous price? "For God *so loved* the world that He gave His only begotten Son, that whoever believes in Him should not

---

[199] Matthew 27:25

perish but have everlasting life."[200] Praise God that He loves us so much!

The Worth of a Soul

So, how much are you worth? You are worth the life of Christ! Why are you worth the life of Christ? Because He was willing to pay that price for you. And why was He willing to pay that price for you? Because He knew you *are* worth the price He paid for you. You see, God doesn't pay for trash. He pays exactly what it is worth.

It was a patient of mine that helped me to understand this concept more clearly. He was dying of cancer, and I was treating him at the end of his life. And while I was trying to be a blessing to him, he was a blessing to me. The following concept came from him.

How many people have there been on this planet since Adam and Eve until now? Let us just imagine that it is 20 billion people. What is the average lifespan of people from creation until now? Most people before the flood lived over 900 years, but there have been many children since who died shortly after birth. Let us say that the average life span is 100 years. So, 20 billion people living an average of 100 years would then represent 2 trillion human life-years.

And what has been accomplished in the last 6,000 years by 20 billion people over 2 trillion life-years? See the advancements that have been made, books written, devices developed, infrastructure constructed, etc.

Now, take one person and give them eternal life. When Jesus comes, they are resurrected and go with Him to heaven. They live 1,000 years, 2,000 years, and 5,000 years. They live 10,000 years, 100,000 years and a million years. They live 2 million, then 5 million, then 10 million. They live 100 million, a billion, 10 billion and 100 billion. They live a trillion years and then 2 trillion years. Then they

---

[200] John 3:16

live 3 trillion years, 5 trillion, 100 trillion, a quadrillion, quintillion, sextillion, septillion, octillion, nonillion and decillion years.

Eventually, a single individual, saved in eternity, will accomplish infinitely more than all that humanity has accomplished since creation until now. God knew what you were worth, and He paid the price that you were worth.

Treat It Like It's Worth It

Let us imagine that we have two vases. One is from Walmart and costs $1. The other is Ming Dynasty, and is worth $3,500,000. Would you treat each of the vases the same? They both have the same function. They are both vases. They both can hold water or marbles or plants or other things. They can both the placed in the middle of the table to hold something beautiful or interesting to look at. But, while they both have the same function, their value is significantly different.

Would you put water and flowers in the Ming Dynasty vase? Would you carry it around the house over your tile floors? Would you clean it in the sink like you do the Walmart vase? Would you leave the flowers to rot in it? Would you leave it on the edge of the book shelf where it could possibly be knocked off? No! You wouldn't do any of those things.

You would protect the Ming Dynasty vase. You wouldn't put anything inside of it. You probably wouldn't touch it without gloves on your hands. You would make sure that if it is ever moved, it is done with utmost care and caution. You would probably keep it in a prominent place where there would be virtually no possibility of it falling and breaking.

Something's perceived value determines how you treat it. What is your value? You are worth the life of Christ. So, how should you treat yourself? You should treat yourself like you're worth the price He paid for you.

If you are worth the life of Christ, shouldn't that change how you treat yourself? Shouldn't that change what you eat and drink? Shouldn't that change how you dress and speak? Shouldn't that change how you exercise and rest? Shouldn't that change how you think and act?

"Or do you not know that your body is the temple of the Holy Spirit who is in you, whom you have from God, and you are not your own? For you were bought at a price; therefore glorify God in your body and in your spirit, which are God's."[201] "Therefore, whether you eat or drink, or whatever you do, do all to the glory of God."[202]

How much are others worth? Regardless of their situation in life or how degraded they have become through poor choices and difficult circumstances; every human being is worth the life of Christ. And if that is so, how will you treat them? You will treat them according to the value that they have in Christ. You will love them, respect them, treat them well, and sacrifice for their restoration.

"The value of a soul, who can estimate? Would you know its worth, go to Gethsemane, and there watch with Christ through those hours of anguish, when He sweat as it were great drops of blood. Look upon the Saviour uplifted on the cross. Hear that despairing cry, "My God, My God, why hast Thou forsaken Me?" Mark 15:34. Look upon the wounded head, the pierced side, the marred feet. Remember that Christ risked all. For our redemption, heaven itself was imperiled. At the foot of the cross, remembering that for one sinner Christ would have laid down His life, you may estimate the value of a soul."[203]

---

[201] 1 Corinthians 6:19,20
[202] 1 Corinthians 10:31
[203] White, E.G. (1900). Christ's Object Lessons. (p. 196). Review and Herald Publishing Association.

CHAPTER TWELVE

A Love that Surrenders

4. Surrender My Life Entirely to Him
The Wheelbarrow

O
n June 30, 1859, about 25,000 people gathered to watch French acrobat and tightrope walker, Charles Blondin, attempt to cross Niagara Falls. As this particular version of the story goes, Blondin first attempted to cross the falls with his 50lb balancing pole, successfully passing from America to Canada. Next, he attempted to cross back to America, using only his arms to balance. Next, he came back across pushing a wheelbarrow in front of him. Then he went out on the line and juggled while he walked. For a grand finale, he did a flip and successfully landed on the line.

The crowd, however, wanted more. So Blondin thought for a while and came up with a plan. He would put someone in the wheelbarrow and push them across the falls to the other side. The crowd cheered at the idea. Then Blondin called to the crowd, asking for a volunteer. Everything went silent. No one volunteered.

Jesus has made it safely across the chasm of sin. He has proved that He can do it. We have proved that we cannot. The only way we are going to get across is if He takes us across. He offers to bring us across (grace), knowing that we cannot make it ourselves. But in order to take us across, we have to exercise faith. Faith is not standing on the ground, looking up at Jesus and saying, "Yes, I believe you can get me across." Faith is *getting into* the wheelbarrow. And that is absolutely terrifying! You see, when you are in the wheelbarrow, you have absolutely no control.

I remember when I was challenged with this decision. I had grown up in church, but I had some addictions that I couldn't overcome. My life began spinning out of control, and I found myself on the verge of leaving my family and plunging into my addictions without restraint. At that point, I was confronted, and challenged to give God another try. I thought I had "tried" God before, but this time I was challenged to give up all control of my life. For the first time in my life, I found myself in a situation that I couldn't get out of, and I realized that I had no answers. I was destroying my life and hurting my loved ones, and if I continued on my current course, I was going to kill myself.

I was challenged to "get into the wheelbarrow." I realized that if I was to make that decision, I would no longer have control of my life. Figuratively, I looked God in the eye at that moment and said, "I don't know if I can trust you. I know you want me to get into the wheelbarrow, but I don't know if I can trust you to not drop me." God reminded me that I was inevitably going to destroy myself if I continued to be in control, and that with Him there was a chance of success. So, I made the decision. No matter what You ask me to do, I will do it. No matter what You ask me to stop, I will stop it. No matter what You ask me to give up, I will give it up. If You want my entertainment, You can have it. If You want my thoughts, You can have them. If You want my reputation, You can have it. If You want anything...You can have it. Just save me from this mess!

It was only when I "got into the wheelbarrow" that I began to successfully overcome. It was only then that I could successfully take of God's love, so that it became mine. What about you? What are you struggling with? What have you never been able to overcome? Isn't it time for you to get into the wheelbarrow? You can't make it on your own. You need Him. Won't you make the decision to give Him everything and get into the wheelbarrow? I can tell you from my experience, it is well worth getting into the wheelbarrow. God won't drop you.

By the way, there are two ways that you can ride in the wheelbarrow once you get in. Either you can be stiff, rigid, clinging to the wheelbarrow in a fearful attempt to remain still so you don't tip over. Or, you can relax and enjoy the ride. I recommend you relax. He knows what He is doing and can get you safely across. Enjoy the ride.

Land of Defeat   Pray Bible Serve Obey | Pray Bible Serve Obey   **Land of Victory**

Getting into the Wheelbarrow

Growing up, I struggled to overcome self and sin. I struggled with several addictions, and while I liked the idea of serving God and obtaining heaven, I just couldn't seem to overcome. I did grow up going to church, so I would read in my Bible about people who were victorious in their lives. I read about Enoch, Noah, Abraham, Joseph, Moses, and Daniel. I read about Peter, Paul, Timothy, and Luke. I went to church with people who appeared to be victorious in their personal lives, and I wanted that victory. And as I contemplated their victorious lives, I saw that there were common themes in their lives.

People living in the land of victory would pray. People in the land of victory would read scripture. People in the land of victory would serve others. And people in the land of victory would obey God. Observing their lives and wanting to be victorious myself, I thought, "If the people who are victorious pray, read scripture, serve, and obey, then if I want to overcome, I must pray, read scripture, serve, and obey."

So, I started on my journey from the land of defeat to the land of victory. I would pray. I would read my Bible. I would get involved in service projects. And I would try to obey. But with every attempt to get into the land of victory, I would always fail. It seemed to me like there was a thin, transparent, dividing line between myself and my attempts to overcome and those who were living victorious lives. I couldn't really see the difference between the two, and it frustrated me that I couldn't overcome. I began to think that I was just a defective model. "It works for others, but it doesn't work for me." "Maybe I'm predestined to failure and being loss." "Maybe I've already committed the unpardonable sin, and there's no hope for me." All of these thoughts and more confronted me as I tried to overcome.

What I didn't realize at that time, but which I came to understand later, was that the difference between the attempt to overcome by prayer, scripture reading, service, and obedience, and the life of victory which included prayer, scripture reading, service and obedience, was not a thin, transparent dividing line. It was a vast canyon—a canyon so large and deep and treacherous and wide that no one could possibly get across.

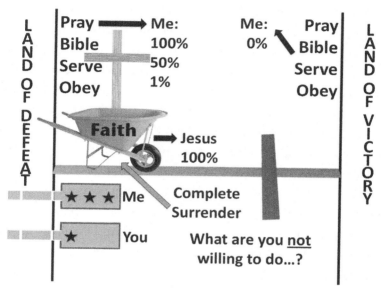

On the other side of this vast canyon in the land of victory, people prayed earnestly and with faith. They read their Bibles and loved what they read. They were naturally involved in serving others. And they obeyed the Lord joyfully.

But over the in land of defeat, there was a different experience. In the land of defeat, it was like I was practicing for the long jump (I used to compete in the long jump in high school). The first time I tried the long jump, I didn't do so well. But as I practiced, my technique improved, and I could jump farther. And as I exercised and built up strength and agility, and as I honed my technique more, I could jump a little farther and a little farther.

So, in the land of defeat I practiced so that I could jump over into the land of victory. I would pray. I would read scripture. I would participate in service projects. And I would try to obey, all in an attempt to get over into the land of victory. And if it didn't work, I would try again. Maybe I would learn a different way to pray or I would learn different ways to study scripture. I would sign up for international mission trips. And I would try and try to obey.

And then I would look around and realize that there are other people who are doing the same thing. Imagine that I had been practicing the long jump for a long time and I can jump pretty far. But you haven't been at it very long, and you can't jump very far. I could look at you and think to myself, "Look at you. You aren't doing so well. I'm so much better than you are." And in my pride, I could be just like the Pharisee and the tax collector in Luke 18:10-14, "Two men went up to the temple to pray, one a Pharisee and the other a tax collector. The Pharisee stood and prayed thus with himself, 'God, I thank You that I am not like other men—extortioners, unjust, adulterers, or even as this tax collector. I fast twice a week; I give tithes of all that I possess.' And the tax collector, standing afar off, would not so much as raise his eyes to heaven, but beat his breast, saying, 'God, be merciful to me a sinner!' I tell you, this man went down to his house justified rather than the other; for everyone who exalts himself will be humbled, and he who humbles himself will be exalted."

Unfortunately, I have found myself in this situation of judgmental attitudes too many times in my life—looking down upon others because they aren't as "good" as I am or don't have the same "good" practices that I do. Paul tells us, "But they, measuring themselves by themselves, and comparing themselves among themselves, are not wise."[204]

How foolish is this?! Both of us are standing on the edge of an impassible canyon, and I think that I'm better than you because I can jump farther. But both of us are going to fall into the depths of the

---

[204] 2 Corinthians 10:12

canyon to our deaths, because neither of us can possibly jump across
the canyon. What does it matter if I can jump a few more feet than
you, if both of us will die when we jump?

As long as I am trusting in anything that I can do—prayer, Bible
study, service, or obedience, I am practicing for and participating in
the long jump. It doesn't matter if I am trusting in myself and these
things 100%, 50%, or even 1%—if I am trusting in myself and my
practice of these things to any degree, I am in long jump mode, and I
will never get across the canyon. The canyon is impassible by my own
efforts.

But Jesus knew this, and that is why He came and lived a perfect
life in human flesh and died the death that we deserve on the cross.
Jesus spanned the canyon with the tightrope of His perfect life to
make a way across the canyon. And He stands at the edge of the
canyon on the tightrope holding a wheelbarrow, inviting you to get in.
That wheelbarrow represents faith—a faith that trusts in Jesus and
surrenders the life to Him.

On the other side, in the land of victory, people pray, read their
Bible, serve, and obey, but they do not trust in these things to get
them across the canyon. There is 0% trust in myself, my prayer, my
Bible reading, my service, my obedience, etc. to get me across. In the
wheelbarrow, there is 100% trust in Jesus to get me across the canyon
to victory.

A question that can be asked at this point is: what are you not
willing to do to be free—to be victorious? Maybe you aren't willing to
give up your entertainment. Maybe you aren't willing to give up your
career. Maybe you aren't willing to give up your friends or family,
because they will reject you if you follow Jesus. Maybe you aren't
willing to give up _____ (you fill in the blank). Whatever
you answer that question with—whatever you are not willing to give up
to be free—is the very thing that will keep you from getting to the

other side. It is the very thing that will keep you from getting to the land of victory.

Getting into the wheelbarrow is an act of faith, and it is potentially one of the most frightening decisions that you and I will make in our lives. Because when we get in the wheelbarrow, we can have no more control of our lives. Jesus has 100% control.

Getting into the wheelbarrow represents complete surrender of myself, my wishes, my desires, my plans, my dreams, my aspirations, and my life to Christ. I am willing to do anything that God asks me to. I am willing to give up anything He asks me to give up. I am willing to face shame, embarrassment, ridicule, suffering, and even death if necessary. I just want to be free. I just want to be victorious. I just want the joy and peace that I have always needed but never possessed with any consistency.

There are two realities that help in this decision. First, if I remain in control of my life and stuck in the land of defeat, I will die and be lost eternally, regardless of whether I go to church (you aren't saved by going to church), profess to be a Christian (I can profess I am a Christian and live like the devil. Profession proves nothing.), or live a "good" life ("There is none who does good, no, not one."[205] "For all have sinned and fall short of the glory of God."[206] "No one is good but One, that is, God."[207] "But we are all like an unclean thing, And all our righteousnesses are like filthy rags...."[208]). I am lost, hopelessly lost, on my own. I cannot save myself. I cannot get to the land of victory on my own.

Second, the land of victory contains everything that I need. There is where perfect love abides. There is where one has and retains peace. There is where perfect joy abides. There is where you find freedom from the past. There is forgiveness for all. There is

---

[205] Romans 3:12
[206] Romans 3:23
[207] Matthew 19:17
[208] Isaiah 64:6

where you become free—truly free. There is heaven. There is eternal life. There is where Jesus abides with and in His people.

You may ask, "How do I get into the wheelbarrow? How do I surrender completely?" Imagine with me that you are holding onto a rope, supporting your entire weight from it. There is no light and no sound. You cannot see or hear anything. You do not know where you are in space in relation to anything else. You try to climb the rope, but there is some ceiling above you that you cannot get around. You come to the end of the rope and stretch as far as you can to see if your toes touch something. They don't. You try swinging from side to side to see if you can feel anything around you that you might be able to grab on to or land on, but you don't find anything.

In this scenario, you can hold on to the rope indefinitely without getting tired and falling off. In fact, you can die holding on to the rope.

Then you hear God's voice say, "Let go of the rope." And you start thinking, "How far is the ground below me? Will I land on flat solid ground? Will it be jagged and rough? Will it be soft and bouncy? Will it be watery and wet? Is it 2 inches below me, 2 feet below me, or 2 miles below me? Will it hurt when I land? Will I die?"

You ask God to answer any or all of these questions, and He gives you no answer. You simply have the request, "Let go of the rope." So, you must ask, "Can I trust myself to God, that when He asks me to let go, it will be okay to let go? Will He take care of the consequences that I do not know about and cannot control? Am I willing to potentially face death and the loss of all things and follow His advice to let go?

You can ask all the questions you want to ask. You can think through all of the scenarios that you want to think through. You can argue with yourself about the cost/benefit ratio of the decision you are asked to make. You can try to intellectually understand everything involved in the process before you let go. But all of this will simply delay your obedience and your freedom. You don't need to figure it out or understand it all. You simply need to obey. You simply need to let go.

Surrender—getting into the wheelbarrow—is not *wanting* to let go. It is not *thinking about* letting go. It is not *agreeing* to let go. It is not even *trying* to let go. Surrender—getting into the wheelbarrow—is simply letting go. And only letting go gets you into the wheelbarrow. Because, when you let go of the rope, you land in the wheelbarrow, and Jesus takes you across the canyon on the tightrope of His perfect life. He makes it work.

"If they would open their hearts fully to receive Christ, then the very life of God, His love, would dwell in them, transforming them into His own likeness; and thus through God's free gift they would possess the righteousness which the law requires."[209]

"All true obedience comes from the heart. It was heart work with Christ. And if we consent, He will so identify Himself with our thoughts and aims, so blend our hearts and minds into conformity to His will, that when obeying Him we shall be but carrying out our own impulses. The will, refined and sanctified, will find its highest delight in doing His service. When we know God as it is our privilege to know Him, our life will be a life of continual obedience. Through an appreciation of the character of Christ, through communion with God, sin will become hateful to us."[210]

Letting go of the rope is taking up your cross and following Christ. "Then He said to them all, 'If anyone desires to come after Me, let him deny himself, and take up his cross daily, and follow Me.'"[211]

---

[209] White, E. G. (1896) *Thoughts from the Mount of Blessing*. (p 54). Mountain View, CA: Pacific Press Publishing Association.
[210] White, E. G. (1898) *The Desire of Ages*. (p 668). Review and Herald Publishing Association.
[211] Luke 9:23

Taking up your cross and following Christ is not about taking up duties and responsibilities that are burdensome and dragging along behind Christ. No! Never! Taking up your cross is about giving up and letting go of the rope. It is about surrendering all of your hopes, wishes, plans, dreams, and aspirations to Christ and letting Him determine the direction and path of your life, whatever may come. Taking up the cross is about surrender.

Jesus wants to accomplish for us things that are infinitely greater than we are looking for ourselves, and in order to do that we must surrender what we want and what we hope for so that He can replace those with His thoughts and plans for us. "'For My thoughts are not your thoughts, nor are your ways My ways,' says the Lord. 'For as the heavens are higher than the earth, so are My ways higher than your ways, and My thoughts than your thoughts.'"[212]

As we surrender entirely to Him, we are grafted into Christ, and we begin to produce His fruit in our lives, for He lives through us. What kind of fruit do we produce? We produce the fruit of the Spirit. "But the fruit of the Spirit is love, joy, peace, longsuffering, kindness, goodness, faithfulness, gentleness, self-control. Against such there is no law."[213] And how many of these fruits will be seen in our lives? Will it only be one or two? No. It will be all of them.

"'Abide in Me, and I in you.' Abiding in Christ means a constant receiving of His Spirit, a life of unreserved surrender to His service. The channel of communication must be open continually between man and his God. As the vine branch constantly draws the sap from the living vine, so are we to cling to Jesus, and receive from Him by faith the strength and perfection of His own character. The root sends its nourishment through the branch to the outermost twig. So Christ communicates the current of spiritual strength to every believer. So long as the soul is united to Christ, there is no danger that it will wither or decay. The life of the vine will be manifest in

---

[212] Isaiah 55:8,9
[213] Galatians 5:22,23

fragrant fruit on the branches. "He that abideth in Me," said Jesus, "and I in him, the same bringeth forth much fruit: for without Me ye can do nothing." When we live by faith on the Son of God, the fruits of the Spirit will be seen in our lives; not one will be missing."[214]

When we are saved by such a loving God and we are released from the failure and misery that our lives have been, won't we express gratefulness to the God who set us free? Won't we live differently than we did before? No longer will we live for ourselves. We will live for Him. No longer will any task or duty be burdensome, because it will be done from love to the One who set us free. We will eat what He created us to eat and drink what He created us to drink and wear what He desires us to wear. We will no longer be a slave to appetite and taste. We will no longer be a slave to fashion and entertainment. We will no longer be a slave to sinful pleasures and earthly powers. We will gladly do what is necessary to keep ourselves in good health, because our bodies are His temple.

When that great salvation becomes ours, we will love those whom He loves and sacrifice ourselves for them, not out of duty, but out of love. We will love what God loves, because He loves it, and we will hate what God hates, because He hates it. Our lives will be entirely transformed, because of love. And in that love, there will be great joy and peace, the ability to suffer long for others, and kindness for others, goodness of life, faithfulness to God, gentleness to all, and self-control.

"If they would open their hearts fully to receive Christ, then the very life of God, His love, would dwell in them, transforming them into His own likeness; and thus through God's free gift they would possess the righteousness which the law requires."[215]

[214] White, E.G. (1898) *The Desire of Ages*. (p 676). Review and Herald Publishing Association.
[215] White, E.G. (1896) *Thoughts from the Mount of Blessing*. (p 54). Mountain View, CA: Pacific Press Publishing Association.

CHAPTER THIRTEEN

A Love that Thinks Well

5. Search my heart

I also spend time searching my heart.

Why do I search my heart? It is because my heart is deceitful, and I don't know what is in it. We each have an amazing capacity to be deceived. We can think we are okay when everything is wrong. And there are at least 3 things that reveal to us, personally, what is in our hearts:

The first thing that reveals to me what is in my heart is trials and my response to them. "Search me, O god, and know my heart; try me, and know my anxieties; and see if there is any wicked way in me, and lead me in the way everlasting."[216] How I respond to a trial reveals to me what is in my heart. The Bible says, "For out of the abundance of the heart the mouth speaks."[217] The way you respond to a trial shows you what was inside your heart in the first place. The reason that it came out was because it was in there. The trial did not cause

---

[216] Psalm 139:23,24
[217] Matthew 12:34

the response, it only elicited the response. The response came because of what was in the heart.

For instance, suppose someone cuts you off on the road and makes a profane gesture at you while speeding away. How do you respond? Anger? Frustration? Pity? Prayer? How you respond is dependent upon what is in your heart. If anger is there, it will come out. If frustration is there, it will come out. If peace is there, it will come out. The trial (your response to it) simply reveals what is in your heart.

A second way that I can know what is in my heart is the body. If I have disease or dysfunction that does not come from inheritance, environment, or raw materials, I can know there is something in my heart. You see, the spirit can be deceived, but the body cannot. The body carries a perfect record of what has been done to it, and the body cannot lie or be deceived. The spirit can, however.

As an analogy, when you write a letter on a piece of paper, does the paper know what you wrote on it? No. Does the paper lie? No. It could be that a lie was written on the paper (by you), but the paper cannot lie. It tells the truth about what was written on it. Similarly, the body does not know what the spirit puts into it. It cannot lie, neither can it be deceived. It simply gives a faithful account of what has been done to it (by the spirit—the heart). So, if the body is diseased or dysfunctional because of "energy" issues (thoughts), you can be sure that the heart has a problem that is manifesting in the body.

And a third way we can know what is in our hearts is our treasure. Matthew 6:21 tells us, "For where you treasure is, there you heart will be also." That which we pursue, that which we spend our time and money on, that which is important to us is our treasure. And that treasure is in the heart. Go through your financial statements and see where your money goes. You'll find your treasure. Make a note of how much time you spend doing X, Y, or Z. You'll find your treasure. Keep a log of what you talk about. You'll find your treasure.

Romans 8:5 tells us, "For those who live according to the flesh set their minds on the things of the flesh, but those who live according to the Spirit, the things of the Spirit."

Determine that every morning you will spend time with God outdoors in nature, just like Jesus did. There is something about being out in nature that attracts you to God and helps you open your heart to Him better than if you were indoors, so I encourage you, get outside in His nature for your prayer time early in the morning, every morning. And if you have children who need you once they wake up, you will need to wake up before them and spend your time with God before they wake up.

In your prayer time, review the previous day's thoughts, words, and actions. Ask God, "What legitimate need of my heart influenced my actions in that situation?" And ask God, "How did my heart deceive me to fulfill that legitimate need in the wrong way?"

I'll give an example to illustrate. One day we were having several committee meetings, and we broke for lunch. After lunch, another committee with many of the same people convened. Wanting to be efficient with our time, I jumped right into our first agenda item. Our vice president kindly stated, "Mr. President, shouldn't we begin with prayer?" Immediately, an excuse came gushing out of my mouth for why I didn't begin with prayer. I asked someone else to pray, and while they were praying, I was thinking, "Lord, why did that excuse just come gushing out of my mouth? I don't understand it. Please remind me tomorrow morning that I want to figure this out."

The following morning, when I was having my walk/talk time with God, I remembered the excuse the previous day, and I asked God, "What was the legitimate need of my heart that drove me to make the excuse?" As I wrestled with God for 15-20 minutes, He finally gave me the answer. That still small voice in my head said, "Mark, you needed acceptance and belonging." In my mind, I responded, "Well, yes, I need acceptance and belonging. But I still don't understand. So, how did my heart deceive me to fulfill my need for acceptance and belonging in the wrong way?" After another 10-15 minutes, God responded, "Mark, you don't need it from them." That's when the light went on. I got it!

"Oh, God, I get it. I thought I needed acceptance and belonging from the other committee members, and when my mistake was pointed out, I needed to make an excuse to mitigate the mistake. The reality is that I don't need acceptance and belonging from them. I only need it from you, so I don't need to make an excuse, because I won't lose acceptance and belonging from you by making a mistake. My acceptance and belonging in you are secure."

Now I understand that part of my heart, and the next time that situation arises, at least I'll know what's going on in my heart. And eventually I'll be able to avoid making an excuse, because I'll remember that God is my only source for acceptance and belonging.

6. Choose to Think Only Positively About Them

We need to think only positively about "them," regardless of what they have done to us. There was a patient that I took care of once who was suffering from severe stomach pain related to gastritis and reflux disease. She had been treated by doctors for years without success and was using natural remedies trying to keep her symptoms under control. When I began seeing her for her symptoms, I quickly discovered that she had a lot of bitterness toward her ex-husband. Every time I would meet with her, her symptoms would improve for hours to a day or so, and then her thinking would get the best of her and her digestive issues would get worse.

I knew that there are more neurons in the digestive tract than the spinal cord, and that issues of the mind have a strong impact on the function of the digestive system. I was convinced that her bitterness toward her ex-husband was a major contributing factor to her disease process, so I gave her a homework assignment to do before our next appointment. I asked her to think of two things that were positive about her ex-husband, write them down, and bring them with her for our next visit. At that next visit, she had zero good things to say about her ex-husband.

At that next visit, I confronted her with the need to think positively about everyone in her life, including her ex-husband. I asked her, "Does God love your ex-husband?"

She said, "Of course He loves my ex-husband. God loves everybody."

"What does God love about your ex-husband?"

"Oh, I don't know what He would love about him...he was such a...." and on, and on she went, recounting the negative qualities of her ex-husband. I gave her another homework assignment to complete before our next appointment. I asked her to ask God in her prayer time, "God, what do you love about my ex-husband?" and write that down and bring it to me at our next appointment. At that next appointment, she had nothing. We had several more appointments, and she never ended up with even one good thing about her ex-husband.

Was she right when she agreed that God does love her ex-husband? Yes. Is her ex-husband without any good qualities? No. There was something that she fell in love with in the first place before she married him. God loves her ex-husband. He loves him enough to die for him. He is interceding on his behalf in heaven right now. He loves him deeply! She had nothing good to say about her ex-husband because she was unwilling to see any good in him. She was unwilling to see him through Jesus' eyes.

Can you guess what happened with her digestive problems? They got worse, not better! And she became bitter toward me later, because I didn't help her condition improve. I am convinced that if she would have yielded to the Lord's leading and would begin to see her ex-husband through Jesus' eyes—if she would choose to think positively about her ex-husband—the bitterness would, by God's grace, go away, and she would begin to see all the others in her life from that same new light—and her digestive issues would resolve!

To think only positively about someone who has hurt you is impossible to accomplish on your own. Only God can accomplish it in your life. So, if you succeed, it is clear evidence that God is working in you. Again, like in the story above, if you have a hard time finding something positive to think about them, ask God, "Why do you love them? Please show me what you see so I can see the same things. Help me to love them like You do." And He will!

Escaping the Bitterness Trap

Let us focus in on bitterness so that we can understand why it is what it is, and so that we can find the right solution for it.

First of all, we understand that there is only one God. "For You are great, and do wondrous things; You alone are God."[218] And God is a just God. He is just because of Who He is, and He manifests His justice for the sake of others, not for His own sake. His justice is selfless, not selfish. "...all His ways are justice, a God of truth and without injustice; righteous and upright is He."[219]

When we sin, the act may have been perpetrated upon others, but the sin is against God and His law. "Against You, You only, have I sinned, and done this evil in Your sight..."[220] "...sin is the transgression of the law."[221] For every law, there is a penalty if it is broken, and the penalty for sin is death. "For the wages of sin is death..."[222]

Because sin is against God and His law, God must be the one to uphold His law, and therefore, He is the one to administer or exact the penalty that the law requires. "'Vengeance is Mine, I will repay,'

[218] Psalm 86:10
[219] Deuteronomy 32:4
[220] Psalm 51:4
[221] 1 John 3:4
[222] Romans 6:23

says the Lord." [223] Only when the penalty is paid in full is justice satisfied and the punishment complete. This is how sin and justice relate in God's government. But what happens in bitterness?

Bitterness stems from our core identity crisis. I believe that I am god. And when you did something that hurt me, you sinned against me. That sin requires a penalty, and I must uphold "justice" by making you pay for what you did. The problem is that my justice is for self's sake—it is motivated by selfishness. I try to extract the penalty from you, and I will only allow you to go free when you have paid the penalty in full. If you do not pay the penalty in full, you will never go free.

I often describe bitterness in relation to a prison cell. You did something to hurt me—you wronged me, so I put you in a prison cell. You will stay in that prison cell until you pay back all that you owe because of the sin you committed against me. The problem is that you cannot pay for what you did, therefore you will never get out of the prison cell I put you in. This is the deception of the bitterness prison.

The reality is that, when you sinned, you wronged God and are ultimately responsible to Him, not me. In thinking that I am God and attempting to put you in the prison cell, I actually put myself in the prison cell, thinking that you are the one inside. I will stay inside the prison cell until you pay everything that you owe me for the sin I believe you committed against me. The problem is that you cannot pay for what you did, so I will never get out of the prison cell I locked myself in. Although I do not realize it, I am my own jailer. This is the horrible reality of bitterness.

In this situation, I must be willing to let you go free if I am going to be able to go free. But I will not let you go free, because if I let you go without paying your debt, my sense of "justice" will not be satisfied. In other words, you will get away with it. And if I cannot

---

[223] Romans 12:19

allow you to go free, I will never go free, because it is me who is locked inside the prison cell, not you.

There is a key that can open this prison cell, and that key is forgiveness. Ironically, I remain locked inside the prison cell while holding the key in my hand. I refuse to use the key, because, in my deception, I fear that if I use the key, you will go free.

I try to hold you to my hurt feelings until you suffer enough to pay for your sin, but no measure of suffering can undo the past. And regardless, no one is so hurt by my hurt feelings as I am. So, if I try to hold you to my hurt feelings so that you hurt for what you did, I do most or all of the suffering, while you do less to none of it. Again, since you cannot pay for what you did, I will remain captive forever. If I let go of the hurt feelings, you go free, and I don't want you to go free until you have paid everything you are supposed to pay. So, I hold on to the hurt feelings in an attempt to keep you captive—in order to exact justice. This, friends, is the foundation of bitterness. And it is ugly.

Not only are we deceived when it comes to bitterness, but the Christian world is deceived when it comes to forgiveness as well. The "Christian" understanding of forgiveness goes like this: You hurt me somehow (you sinned against me), and because of what you did, you must pay. But I choose to set you free, to remit your debt, to not make you pay for what you did. Therefore, I forgive you. But in this familiar scenario, I approach forgiveness from the standpoint of god. You sinned against me. You owe me. I set you free. I am still god, but this cannot be.

The proper foundation for forgiveness is the understanding that I am not god. What you did to me was really against God. Your debt is to Him, not me.

I came to the cross and accepted the divine exchange on my behalf, and in so doing, Jesus took my place. He became the victim for me. And what you did to me is now what you did to Jesus. I am no longer the victim, because Jesus took my place and became the victim for me. I go free. You owe me nothing. Your debt is to God. And the same God who set me free at the cross is the same God who can set you free at the cross. In accepting His love for me at the cross, I now have love for you, and I want to see God set you free just like He set me free. And if I can do anything to help in the process of your freedom, I am happy to do so, even if it is a sacrifice on my part. This is the true foundation for forgiveness. This is the true solution for bitterness. And it is found only at the cross.

How do I know when I have truly resolved my bitterness through forgiveness? I will still remember what happened, but the memory will no longer be painful. I can think about it without pain, anger, bitterness, or shame. Why? Because God has healed the hurt by His healing grace. He sets me free.

Feeling Guilty

If I confess my sins, You are faithful and just to forgive me my sins, and to cleanse me from all unrighteousness.
– 1 John 1:9

Thank you, Lord, for giving me the truth of Your Word. I **choose** to believe that I am forgiven, because you said so. Thank you for forgiving me!

Overcoming Negative Thoughts

When we try to overcome negative thinking and negative thinking patterns, it helps to understand the Displacement Principle. To understand the displacement principle, we need to understand a little bit more of how the mind was created to operate.

First of all, the mind was created to be occupied. It wasn't created to be a void. There is no admonition in scripture for the mind to be emptied or for us to meditate by emptying our mind. We are admonished, "Let this mind be in you which was also in Christ Jesus." [224] "Meditate [think] upon these things." [225] "Occupy till I come." [226] There is an example given in the Bible about what happens when there is empty space. In Matthew 12:43-45 the example is given of a man who has a demon cast out of him. The demon leaves him alone for a while, but then comes back later and "finds it empty, swept, and put in order." He then gets seven other demons, worse than himself, and they all come and possess the man, who is worse off than he was at the beginning. In short, the enemy occupies empty space.

Please don't get fooled here. I have been involved in apparently "Christian" meditation practices where I tried to empty my mind of all thoughts so that God could speak to me. In the quiet, I heard the words, "Mark, I love you." At first, I thought it was my own thoughts, but eventually I believed that it was God speaking to me. I felt such love that my spirit so badly needed. But in time, I began to trust in that "Jesus" and his voice in my head. I would make decisions based upon what he would "tell" me, and I made some really big mistakes. When I finally looked back at the situation, I realized that it was the enemy that was leading me, imperceptibly, down a pathway to destruction.

Satan was in heaven. He knows what heaven's love feels like, and he can reproduce it very well. It felt good. It looked good. But I began to spend much more time with that "Jesus" and less and less time with my Bible. I began to trust the "voice" in my head and stopped reading the only book that could show me my danger—the Bible.

Healthy meditation is not emptying one's mind so that God can speak to you. Healthy meditation is thinking about His promises,

---

[224] Philippians 2:5
[225] Philippians 4:8
[226] Luke 19:13

reading His word, contemplating His life and love, and the mansions He is preparing for us. Healthy meditation is filling the mind with God's word and contemplating His life. The mind was created to be occupied.

But while the mind must be occupied, it is limited in that it can only focus on one thing at a time. I don't care how good of a multi-tasker you are; you cannot focus on two things at one time. That's why in many states it is illegal for you to text while driving.

Because the mind was created to be occupied, you and I cannot overcome negative thoughts simply by trying to not think about the negative thoughts. Why? It is trying to create a void—to empty the mind which was created to be occupied. It doesn't work. The entire time that you are trying to not think about the negative thought, you are thinking about the negative thought. But this is the main thing we do when we try to not think about a negative thought, and this is why we fail at overcoming the negative thoughts.

But the second principle of the mind—that the mind cannot focus on more than one thing as the same time—is the key to overcoming the negative thoughts. If I actively think about or focus on something else, I cannot be thinking about the negative thought at the same time. So, I displace the negative thought with something else, something positive. This is the Displacement Principle.

Let us take a living example of some negative thinking and how the Displacement Principle works. I come from a background of addiction, and one thing that an addict eventually believes is, "I can't do it. I can't overcome. I have tried and tried and failed and failed. It may work for others, but it doesn't work for me. I don't know why I keep on trying. I might as well give up."

Is that a truth or a lie? It is a lie. What does the Bible say? "I can do all things through Christ who strengthens me."[227] So, the truth of God's word is, I can do it. I can overcome through Christ. I don't

___
[227] Philippians 4:13

have to remain a failure. There is help sufficient for me. So, what do I do about it practically? How do I apply this Displacement Principle in real life?

If I have the thought or feeling, "I can't do it." I can write on a 3X5 card, "I *can* do all things through Christ who strengthens me. Philippians 4:13," along with a simple prayer of faith, "Thank you, Lord, for giving me the truth of Your Word. I choose to believe that I *will* overcome, because you said so. Thank you for helping me overcome."

Every time I have the negative thought or feeling of "I can't do it," I take out my 3X5 card and read *out loud* the verse and prayer ("So then faith comes by hearing, and hearing by the word of God."[228]), concentrating on what I am saying. I may still have the thought or feeling after reading the card, but while I was concentrating on the text and prayer, I couldn't have the negative thought also, because I can only focus on one thing at a time.

If the thought comes back, I do it again, and again, and again, until the negative thought or feeling is not there anymore, or I am distracted by something else that needs my attention. And if the thought comes back at some other time, I pull the card back out and start again!

You see, it's like you are in a battle. This is an old-fashioned battle, where the enemy is lined up over there with swords, axes, and spears. And you are over here with your fellow soldiers. As the enemy advances and engages in battle, if you leave your sword in its sheath, what will happen to you? You will die! What if you take your sword out and take one whack at the enemy and then put it back in its sheath? What will happen to you? You will still die. The only way you will live is if you use your sword every time the enemy advances.

Ephesians 6:17 tells us that "the sword of the Spirit...is the word of God." Most Christians fail, not because they don't have the sword,

---

[228] Romans 10:17

not because they haven't memorized some of the sword, but because they fail to properly use the sword. We must use the sword *every time* the enemy advances. Only then will we have victory over the enemy.

In giving in to the negative thoughts over and over again in the past, we have created strong neural pathways in our brains. It is easy for us to go back to the old path, because we have developed strong brain connections that promote that thinking. It is like being in the jungle and having a well-worn pathway. It is available, unobstructed, easy to follow, and familiar. But, in taking up the Sword of the Spirit and choosing to think a different way, you are beginning to cut a new pathway in the jungle.

At the beginning it is very difficult. You have to cut and cut and cut, because there are so many vines and bushes and obstacles in your way. And your forward progress is slow. Your brain needs to develop new connections. There is dendritic branching, and new synaptic connections that develop in the brain. As you continue with the new thinking, the new path becomes easier and easier to go down. In time, the new path becomes the "easy" path.

I remember the first time I realized this in my life. With my addiction, there were some thoughts—negative thoughts—that were always in my head. I didn't know I could go a minute without this stuff going through my head. But, when I began using my 3X5 cards to overcome my negative thoughts, the battle was really hard! It seemed that I needed to use them all the time. I didn't know if I would have time to live life, work, or get anything else done, but I persevered.

I remember about 2-3 months into this process of using the Displacement Principle, that my wife and I were reviewing our day together at the end of the day, and I realized something wonderful. I hadn't had a single one of those thoughts the entire day! Wow! Before, I couldn't get them out of my head for less than a minute.

Now, I went a whole day without even one of those thoughts! I was so excited. I was finding out for myself that it works!

The battles were not over at that point. I still had many months of battles before me, but I could see the victory, and that gave me courage to continue on.

Something else that I discovered later is that dreams lag several years behind the conscious life. When I was overcoming the negative thoughts in my conscious life, I would still be plagued by bad dreams—like I was back in my addiction. But several years after overcoming in my conscious thoughts, my dreams began to "clear up," and match my conscious experience. Praise the Lord!

Now, here are a couple points that I need to make. First of all, I only recommend that you carry with you three 3X5 cards or fewer. I have seen this method fail with people who have many different Bible promises written down. If you are in a battle, and you have hundreds of weapons to choose from, you may be killed by the enemy before you ever choose which weapon you will use in the attack. Keep it simple, know your weapons well, use them often, and you will be an effective and efficient soldier.

With your 3X5 cards, I recommend you follow the 4-Second Rule. The 4-Second Rule is this: once you realize that you are thinking a negative thought, you have 4 seconds to pull out your 3X5 card and begin reading out loud your text and prayer of faith. You may have been thinking about the negative stuff for minutes or even hours without being aware of what you were doing, but once you become aware of it, you have 4 seconds to pull out your card and read.

Another lie that I, and many others, have accepted is, "I am unloved." But what does the Bible say? "I have loved you with an everlasting love; therefore with lovingkindness I have drawn you."[229]

---

[229] Jeremiah 31:1

Every time you feel that you are unloved, pull out your 3X5 card and recite, "I have loved you with an everlasting love, therefore with lovingkindness I have drawn you. Jeremiah 31:3. Thank you, Lord, for giving me the truth of your word. I choose to believe that I am loved, because you said so. Thank you for loving me." Again, every time the feeling or thought comes, respond with the Word of God, and you will overcome more and more each day.

Another thing we suffer from is guilt. I can have a good or bad response to guilt. A good response to guilt is to see that the guilt is specific to a particular sin, and my response is to confess that sin and repent and go to God for forgiveness. A bad response to guilt is to be caught up in a general sense of guilt without it being tied to a specific sin or sins, and letting that guilt separate me from God because I feel guilty and don't want to come to God and bother Him with my continued failures.

If I have guilt from specific sins, I should confess those sins to God and to those who were hurt through them. If the sin was private, then I confess it privately to God alone. If the sin affected my family, I confess that sin to my family. If the sin is generally known to the entire church, then I confess before the entire church.

Then there is repentance that is needed. What is repentance? "Repentance includes sorrow for sin, and a turning away from it."[230] Repentance is a gift of God and cannot be generated by you and me. We must seek for it from God. And true repentance will always turn away from sin.

Guilt is another negative thought/emotion that I struggled with for years. That guilt led me to despair, thinking that I have been too bad to be forgiven. Let me tell you personally, life is miserable when you feel like that. But is it true that I have been too bad to be forgiven?

---

[230] White, E. G. (1892) *Steps to Christ*. (p. 23). Mountain View, CA: Pacific Press Publishing Association.

But what does the Bible say? "If we confess our sins, He is faithful and just and will forgive us our sins, and cleanse us from ALL unrighteousness."[231]

If I am guilty, or if I feel guilty, I can use God's Word to overcome. I can make my 3X5 card and every time the thought or feeling of guilt comes, recite out loud, "If I confess my sins, You are faithful and just to forgive me my sins, and to cleanse me from all unrighteousness. 1 John 1:9. Thank you, Lord, for giving me the truth of Your word. I choose to believe that I am forgiven, because you said so. Thank you for forgiving me!" I can choose with all my being to believe what I am saying. I can tell you from personal experience, if you put your heart and soul into overcoming like this, it works!

Deep Sea Diving

I was a good deep sea diver. God tells us that He "will cast all our sins Into the depths of the sea."[232] I would ask God to forgive me for the sin I committed, but then I would still feel guilty, so I would (figuratively) swim to the bottom of the sea and bring my sin back up to God and ask Him to forgive me again for the same sin. And I would do this over and over again, because I felt guilty.

What I didn't realize at the time was that God's forgiveness of me does not depend upon how I feel. It depends upon God's word and my complying with the conditions of forgiveness (confession, repentance, restitution).

Penance

Sometimes we are really good at penance. You know what penance is, right? It is where you beat yourself up for the sins that you have committed. Some people actually beat themselves and go on painful pilgrimages in order to atone for their sin. But there is only

[231] 1 John 1:9
[232] Micah 7:19

one atonement for sin, and that is the Blood of Jesus. What was my form of penance? I would commit a sin, and then I would feel bad about it and beat myself up with guilt over it for a while, and when I felt like I had beat myself up enough, I would then accept God's forgiveness. But the whole time I was beating myself up, I was paying penance for my sins, trying to save myself by my own works. This never works. You can come to Jesus in the midst of your sin, accept His forgiveness for you right then and there, and turn away from that sin.

<u>Thought Journal</u>

If you have many different negative thoughts running through your head, and you don't know what texts to use, I recommend that you keep a thought journal for a few days.

Simply carry the journal (it can be as simple as a piece of paper) with you for several days, and write down every negative thought that you have. Next, categorize the negative thoughts. They may fit under *fear/worry*, or feeling *unloved*, or *failure/defeat*, or *guilt/shame*, or *lack of worth/inadequacy*, or *bitterness/anger*, etc. After you have categorized all of your negative thoughts, find the 3 categories which are either the most distressing to you, or which occupy most of your thinking time.

Then go through the Bible (it helps to use a Bible concordance, an online Bible, or a friend to help you) and find promises that speak to your heart the opposite of what the negative thought category is. Write one promise down on your 3X5 card as well as a prayer of faith which goes something like this: "Lord, thank you for giving me the truth of Your word. I choose to believe _____ (Fill in whatever the Bible promise is telling you. For example, I choose to believe that I will overcome...I choose to believe that I am loved...I choose to believe I am forgiven...I choose to believe I have nothing to fear...I choose to believe I am worth the price you paid for me...)

because You said so. Thank You for _____ (Fill in whatever the Bible promise is telling you. For example, Thank You for...helping me overcome...loving me...forgiving me...being with me...giving me such worth...).

The Direction of Your Life

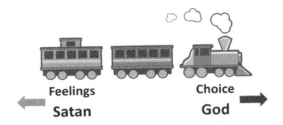

What direction is your life headed in? Our lives are kind of like a train. The train should be driven by the engine, which represents choice. And at the end of the train comes one's feelings. God drives the train of your life by securing your choices. And that moves you in the right direction, as those choices are submitted to God.

Satan, however, tries to drive your train backwards by manipulating your feelings. By manipulating your feelings and making you feel one way or the other, he tries to get your choices. And when he can manipulate you by your feelings in order to get your choices, he can drive your life in the direction he wants you to go in. Don't live as a slave to your feelings. Follow God by choice, regardless of how you feel.

The Law of the Mind

There is a law by which your mind operates. And this law is highlighted by Paul, "But we all, with unveiled face, beholding as in a mirror the glory of the Lord, are being transformed into the same image...."[233] Stated in a simple way, this law says, "By beholding we become changed."

However hateful it is to you, you become like what you concentrate upon. Conversely, as we behold the lovely and the good, we cannot help but becoming like what we behold. This means we have the obligation to choose what we think about, because it will change (literally) who we are.

"It is a law both of the intellectual and the spiritual nature that by beholding we become changed. The mind gradually adapts itself to the subjects upon which it is allowed to dwell. It becomes assimilated to that which it is accustomed to love and reverence."[234]

"Brethren and sisters, it is by beholding that we become changed. By dwelling upon the love of God and our Saviour, by contemplating the perfection of the divine character and claiming the righteousness of Christ as ours by faith, we are to be transformed into the same image. Then let us not gather together all the unpleasant pictures—the iniquities and corruptions and disappointments, the evidences of Satan's power—to hang in the halls of our memory.... There are, thank God, brighter and more cheering pictures which the Lord has presented to us. Let us group together the blessed assurances of His love as precious treasures, that we may look upon them continually."[235]

Senses vs. Feelings

Let us for a moment separate senses and feelings. Sensation includes the physical senses of sight, hearing, smell, taste, and touch. These are your inputs. This is how the physical world impacts your mind.

---

[233] 2 Corinthians 3:18
[234] White, E. G. (1911). *The Great Controversy.* (p 554). Pacific Press Publishing Assn., California.
[235] White, E. G. (1988). *Lift Him Up.* (p 251). Review & Herald Publishing Assn., Maryland.

Feelings, however, are emotional states or reactions to the senses and thoughts that an individual experiences. These are your outputs. This is how you respond and how you feel in responding. You cannot control the reception of a stimulus. If you hit your finger with hammer, you will sense pain. But you can control your feelings—your emotional reactions to those sensations or perceptions. For example, if you hit your finger with a hammer, it will cause pain. But you don't have to get angry because of it. You can be thankful to God that the injury wasn't any worse than it was. You can control your responses by God's power.

In controlling the inputs, we must consider how much time and interest and effort and money we are spending on the best, versus how much time and interest and effort and money we are spending on the rest. How much time do you spend in study of scriptures, reading devotional material, prayer, helping others, or contemplating the love of God?

Compared to that, how much time do you spend watching TV, movies, YouTube, or the news; browsing through Facebook, Twitter, Instagram, or other net media; reading novels, magazines, and other uninspired literature; listening to worldly music; catering to the desires of self or getting lost in work; or contemplating your problems, the pleasures of the world, your faults or those of others, or worrying about things? It is within your capacity, by God's grace, to control your environment such as to avoid negative or hurtful inputs.

"Finally, brethren, whatever things are true, whatever things are noble, whatever things are just, whatever things are pure, whatever things are lovely, whatever things are of good report, if there is any virtue and if there is anything praiseworthy—meditate on these things."[236]

But we can also control the outputs. You are not a slave to your feelings. You can choose how you will respond. Cheerfulness is a

---

[236] Philippians 4:8

choice, not just the result of cheerful circumstances. Thankfulness is a choice, not the result of good things happening to you. We are instructed, "in everything give thanks; for this is the will of God in Christ Jesus for you."[237] If it were not possible, God would not require it of us.

"A life in Christ is a life of restfulness. There may be no ecstasy of feeling, but there should be an abiding, peaceful trust. Your hope is not in yourself; it is in Christ. Your weakness is united to His strength, your ignorance to His wisdom, your frailty to His enduring might. So you are not to look to yourself, not to let the mind dwell upon self, but look to Christ. Let the mind dwell upon His love, upon the beauty, the perfection, of His character. Christ in His self-denial, Christ in His humiliation, Christ in His purity and holiness, Christ in His matchless love—this is the subject for the soul's contemplation. It is by loving Him, copying Him, depending wholly upon Him, that you are to be transformed into His likeness."[238]

So, what about you? Will you trust in God? Will you bring all of your thoughts into captivity to His will? Will you replace those negative thoughts with the truth of His word and overcome by His power?

As you go through the painful process of forgiveness, as you go through the arduous task of taking *every* thought captive to the obedience of Christ, as you struggle in the Strength of the Lord until you are successful, be hopeful and faithful, because "He who promised is faithful."[239] He will not disappoint you. It may seem like an impossible task, but God is the God of the impossible.

---

[237] 1 Thessalonians 5:18
[238] White, E. G. (1892) *Steps to Christ*. (p 70). Mountain View, CA: Pacific Press Publishing Association.
[239] Hebrews 10:23

CHAPTER FOURTEEN

A Love that Gives All

7. Love Others

We need to treat them with Love. We need to think about them lovingly. We need to speak to them with love in our voice. We need to treat them with love, choosing to sacrifice ourselves for them and their best good. And this is what happens when the Holy Spirit is living out His life within us, when we are operating with God's heart of divine love. We can seek to be a conduit of God's love to them. Again, we don't create love, only God does. So, we need to come to Him to take from Him of His love, so that it can flow through us to others.

It helps us to remember that they hurt Jesus, not us. When we come to the cross and accept the divine exchange on our behalf, it becomes God's past and we are set free from that burden, that baggage. And just like someone who is ministering to prison inmates in prison ministries, we can love them, because they didn't do it to me. They did it to Jesus.

To highlight what true love looks like, I quote Mark Finley, "In the early 1990's, one of the most horrible events in the history of the world occurred—the genocide in Rwanda. In that genocide—Hutu's battling against Tutsi's—a million people were killed in less than nine months. When the genocide began, there were 370,000 Seventh-day Adventists in Rwanda. When it ended, 100,000 were dead. In six months, 100,000 Adventists were slain, not because they were Adventist, but because they were a part of the minority tribe.

In recent years, I have traveled to Rwanda on a number of occasions speaking in large stadiums. There are trials going on right now trying the killers. As we traveled there, I talked to my host, the Union President, Aman Rutilinga, and I said, 'Pastor Rutilinga, did anyone you know die in the genocide?'

He said, 'Pastor Mark, I was out preaching the day that the radio announcement came, 'Cut down the tall trees,' and when the radio announcement came, 'Cut down the tall trees,' tens of thousands of militia, largely young people with machetes ran through the streets killing every Tutsi they could see. The killing was so great that the bodies stacked up in the streets and dogs came and ate them. The killing was so great that they threw thousands of bodies into the river, and the river was clogged with bodies.'

Pastor Rutilinga was out preaching as Union President, the militia came into the church [and] brought out his wife, his children, and his three grandchildren and killed them outside the church that day.

I talked to the Conference President, 'Did you lose anybody?'

He said, 'Yes I did.'

I said, 'Who did you lose?'

He said, 'I lost my wife and my seven children.'

I talked to my driver, 'Did you lose anybody?'

'Yeah. I lost 47 members of my family. I'm the only one that survived.'

As I talked to them, Pastor Aman Rutilinga said to me, 'Mark, I want you to meet a woman, and when you meet her, your life will be changed forever. Her name is Adelle Selfu.'

So we got in the truck and we went on this rough road, back country, outside of Kigali, Rwanda. And Pastor Rutilinga told me the story as we went. This woman had been with her husband when the killers came, and she held his hand as they [used] a machete [to] split his head open, and as they hit him in the neck, and they murdered him. She was there. And Pastor Aman Rutilinga said, 'Mark, I believe she will tell you the story.'

As I walked into her house, I saw a picture of her Seventh-day Adventist pastor husband on the wall, and in respect I simply walked over and stood and looked at the picture. And I thought about what it would be like if I were holding my wife's hand, and someone ran to me and the horror that she would go through as they split my head open with a machete.

As we sat down, we made small talk for a while, and Mrs. Selfu came into the room. And I broached the subject very carefully. I said, 'Sister Selfu, I understand you were with your husband when the militia hacked him to death. It may be very difficult to talk about it, but would you like to share it with me?'

She began to cry, and she said, 'Pastor, I'll share it. We got word that the militia was coming closer and closer to our village. We fled with 45 others to a Catholic church basement. We thought it would be a hiding place. They may go by the church. As we were in the basement, the militia came in with machetes. They began to hack and hack and hack. Actually, there were 60 people in the room. Forty-five were killed immediately.'

She said, 'I held my husband's hand, and someone just came with a machete and hit him in the head, and the blood from his head splat all over me.' She said, 'It was horrible, pastor. And then the person took the machete and hit me in the head.'

She pulled back her beautiful black hair, and I saw a scar that began [at her hair line] and ran down the center of her head. She said, 'Pastor, they then hit me in my wrist, trying to chop off my wrist.' She held up her wrist. It was just flapping around. She said, 'Pastor, then they hit me on the shoulder.' And she pulled down her dress a little bit, and I saw the scar down her shoulder. She said, 'They left me for dead, and my body lay among the dead bodies for three days.

At the end of three days, the militia had moved on, so...villagers came to bury the dead. Somebody, before they buried me, felt my pulse, and I still had a pulse. So, they took me. I was unconscious. They began to nurse me back. Pastor, I was in and out of hospitals for three years.

By this time, the forces that were from outside of Rwanda from the Congo, fought their way back, liberated the country, and they built 18 prisons for the murderers. They put 180,000 people in prison.'

Mrs. Selfu took three years to get back to health, but by now there was stability in the country. And she said to me, 'Pastor Mark, I have to make a decision as to whether I will be a bitter, angry old woman or not.' And she said, 'I made a decision that my husband's death would not be in vain. I had the assurance beating in my heart that Jesus Christ is coming again, and that the thing that my husband would want would be me to go and minister to the killers.

So, Pastor, there is a prison not far from this village, and I became the mother of that prison. I would go in and bring blankets to the prison because [of] the cold nights. I would go in and bring food to the prison. I began studying the Bible with the prisoners. These were killers.

One day, Pastor, I was in the prison. A young man fell at my feet, and he began to kiss my feet. And I looked at his face, and he said, 'Do you remember me?" And she said, 'I wish I could get that face out of my mind. It was the young man in his early 20's who chopped my husband's head in half. It was the young man. I never knew he was in that prison. I never thought that I would see him again. It was the young man who put the scar in my head and gave me such pain. And he said, 'Would you forgive me?'"

And she said, 'I picked him up and I hugged him.' And she said, "I will forgive you.' Pastor, I studied the Bible with him for six months. Pastor, he stood up before the whole prison, and we assembled all the prisoners in the prison yard the day of his baptism, and he confessed his sin. Pastor, we baptized him. Now Pastor, he got amnesty after a few years and was let out of the prison. And here's the problem. His father and mother were killed in the genocide. He had no place to live. Pastor, I adopted him as my son. Would you like to meet him?'

My heart was beating. Beads of perspiration stood [on] my head. I looked at the pastor's picture whom this man had killed. I thought a killer was going to walk through the door, and Luis walked through the door—a gentle smile on his face, a sparkle in his eyes. And Mrs. Selfu walked over, put her arms around him, and she said, 'Let me introduce you to my adopted son.' She said, 'One day when Jesus comes, all the suffering will be worth it all. One day when Jesus comes, all the heartache will be worth it all. One day when Jesus comes, all the burdens will be worth it all. One day when Jesus comes, the past will be gone.' She said, 'What inspires me is the forward look. Jesus is coming again.'"

Is there something in your heart right now that needs to be dealt with? Have you been harboring some bitterness? Is there some sin secretly in your life? If God can transform Adelle Selfu, if God can take that woman and take any bitterness—any anger—out of her heart, God can do miracles in your life.

The Law and the Heart

The Law of Life, taking to give, can only come from a heart that is transformed by the grace of God. It can only come from God's own heart, recreated within us. This Law of Life is in perfect harmony with the 10 commandments, the transcript of God's character. And only one whose heart is operating under the Law of Life, only one whose motive of operation is divine love can keep the law.

If I am living by the old, sinful heart, if I am living under human love—giving to receive, if I am hurt by what others do to me because I am thinking that It's mine, I cannot keep God's law, because His law can only be kept by divine love.

If I try to obey my parents so that I can have long life, I cannot do it with man's heart. If I try to keep my thoughts pure and avoid lustful desires, I cannot do it with man's heart. If I seek to be content with that which I have and not covet that which is my neighbor's, I cannot do it with man's heart. And If I try to keep the Sabbath of the fourth commandment holy, I cannot do it with man's heart.

If we are not on the right side of the equation—if we are not operating with divine love—we cannot keep any of the commandments. It is only by faith in the merits of Christ, it is only faith in His atoning sacrifice, it is only faith that leads to a complete surrender of myself to God that can allow the Holy Spirit to take control of my life and put God's heart within me and give me divine love. With that new heart, I can finally obey the commandments of God, because it is He who is living His life out within me to will and to do of His good pleasure. It is then that sin ceases to be the reality of my life, and I become the righteousness of God.

How can I know which side of the equation I am on? If I think it's mine. If I am hurt personally by what others do. If I give to receive back again, with strings attached, investing with expectation of returns; then all I do amounts to nothing, because I am living by the old, sinful heart. But, if I recognize that it's not mine, that all I have, all I can do, and all I am is God's, if I am not hurt personally by what others do, if I find my joy in giving and I come to God constantly to take from His love so that I can give it to others, if I produce the fruit of God's vine, then I am living by God's heart of divine love.

Love & Liberty

Let us now consider, for a minute, the interrelationship between love and liberty. Human love operates in a predictable manner. As human beings, when we have high interest in someone, we seek to control them more. High interest leads to low freedom (high control). But if we have low interest in someone, we don't try to control them. We give them lots of freedom.

For example, if you are walking down the street and a stranger is smoking a cigarette, you are most likely going to pass on by without a comment. But if it is your 14-year-old child who was smoking, you may walk over to them, grab them by the ear, throw the cigarette on the ground, and take them back home and ground them to their room for a month.

Remember, we must control our sources in order to "protect" our interests—protect our love sources. We do this with God too. There are ways that we try to control Him too. We try to do this or do that, behave this way or behave that way, so that we can manipulate God to do this or that for us. We try to barter with Him, offering Him something (tithe, offerings, time, service, behavior, etc.) in order to get something else in return (forgiveness, acceptance, belonging, security, etc.).

Sometimes, we see Him as the genie in the bottle. If we simply have the right faith—if we rub the bottle the right way—then God will do for us what we wish. Faith, however, is not the hand that moves God to do what I want. It is the hand that accepts from God whatever He sees is best, whether I like it or not.

Divine love operates differently than human love. Divine love maintains maximum interest while at the same time permitting total freedom.

Some of you have probably eaten a Twinkie in the past. Maybe you ate the whole box. Is a Twinkie healthy for you? What about a deep fat fried Twinkie? Is that healthy for you? Absolutely not! And do you know that before you ever try one? Of course, you do.

Does God know it isn't healthy for you? Of course, He does. Does He know that it will contribute to you dying earlier than you would have if you hadn't eaten it? Of course. But does God ever get that Twinkie and knock it out of your hand, grab you by the ear and drag you home and ground you because you were going to eat that Twinkie? Or does He allow you to eat it if you so choose? He allows you to do it.

He loves you infinitely, but He respects your freedom. He will not force you to do good, neither will He prevent you from harming yourself. You can kill yourself quickly or slowly if you choose. He will respect your choice.

He may speak to your conscience and reason with you and try to convince you to change your mind, but He will not force you to do right. You see, love exists in the framework of freedom, and in order for love to be maintained, freedom must be maintained as well. You are not God's source, so He is not dependent upon you. But in order to give you the freedom to love Him in return (because He loves you), He has to give you total freedom to choose Him...or choose something else. Because He loves you so perfectly, He gives you complete freedom to destroy yourself, if you so choose.

God's love—real love—gives perfect liberty to choose the good or the bad. But when you and I attempt to control others, we are operating outside of love. And since we were created in the image of God, we were created to think and act like God, and our body was created to respond perfectly to love. But when we control others, we are operating outside of love, and the result is damage to the soul and the body. We cannot maintain proper function if we are operating outside of the context of love.

And this is true even when we try to control others for the good. We believe something to be right, and we want those whom we love to be right, so we try to control them to do the right so that they can be right. We do it from selfish motives, though. They are our source, and we want them to be a better source for us, so we try to fix them to match what we understand is good. And when they don't respond, we are frustrated and upset, and perhaps we even try to control them in different ways or more forcefully in the future in order to obtain compliance and uniformity. Those we have as the greatest treasures are those whom we try to control the most.

But we also try to control others relative to issues or principles that are dear to us. We will control strangers who are not sources if it is related to an issue or a principle that we are passionate about. Our actions are still from the motive of selfishness, and the result is an attempt to control others.

This selfish, human propensity, when unchecked, will eventually lead us not just to limit the freedom of those who do not comply with our ideas of right, but to destroy them if they refuse to conform to our ideals. This is the foundation of the erosion of religious liberty, and it will be seen more and more clearly in this great country in the next few years. You will see American liberties removed, restrictions imposed, and increasing penalties for nonconformity. And eventually there will be the death penalty for those who will not follow the nation's ideals of right and wrong, even though those ideals are in direct opposition to the Word of God.

Looking back to God and His love and the perfect freedom by which it operates, I am not saying that real freedom can be found in choosing whatever I want and in going in whatever direction I want to go. True freedom is only found in the context of boundaries—the boundaries of God's law.

"True liberty and independence are found in the service of God. His service will place upon you no restriction that will not increase your happiness. In complying with His requirements, you will find a peace, contentment, and enjoyment that you can never have in the path of wild license and sin. Then study well the nature of the liberty you desire. Is it the liberty of the sons of God, to be free in Christ Jesus? or do you call the selfish indulgence of base passions freedom? Such liberty carries with it the heaviest remorse; it is the cruelest bondage."[240]

And looking back to God and His love and the perfect freedom by which it operates, I am not saying that God's love allows evil to happen without consequences. There are consequences. There are always consequences.

It was a divine law that, "whatever a man sows, that he will also reap."[241] And this same law shows us that, "He who sows sparingly will also reap sparingly, and he who sows bountifully will also reap bountifully."[242] There are consequences to the decisions we make.

How does God train His sinful, wayward children? It is not by preventing them from doing wrong. He will teach them, educate them, warn them, reason with them, give them examples of others who have made the same bad decisions; all so that He can give them the best information from which to make their decision. But the decision is theirs. And God will not prevent it. But when the decision is made, there are specific consequences to that decision. And God teaches us through those consequences. They are for the purpose of diverting us from wrong and leading us back to the right.

Remember, He is the Good Shepherd, searching for the lost sheep so that He can lovingly carry it back home. The consequences are not for the purpose of punishment and abandonment. They are for the purpose of redemption and restoration.

In protecting freedom, do we have to eliminate standards? No. God maintains perfect freedom and at the same time holds up

---

[240] White, E.G. (1923) *Fundamentals of Christian Education*. (p. 88). Nashville, TN: Southern Publishing Association.
[241] Galatians 6:7
[242] 2 Corinthians 9:6

definite standards. God gives us freedom to follow or break those standards, but there are consequences for keeping (good consequences) or breaking (bad consequences) those standards.

Every person, family, organization and government must have standards for its members; and those standards must be taught, their obedience encouraged, and their violation enforced. But, mind you, enforcement is through the designated authorities (parents, church board, police, etc.).

Freedom *is not* eliminating the standards or preventing their enforcement. Freedom *is* allowing each individual the liberty to either obey and enjoy the blessings of obedience or disobey and suffer the consequences of disobedience. Each one has the choice to make of whether they will obey or disobey, follow or not follow.

In true freedom, the authority will enforce the consequences of breaking the principle, but they will do so with a selfless motivation. They will enforce the consequences for the benefit of the offender (to motivate them to obey and to limit the burden of sin in the offender's life) as well as the benefit of others (to motivate others to obey by using the offender as an example and protecting others from further, similar violations).

Sin & Grace

There is a relationship between sin and grace that maybe we haven't thought much of. We sin by God's grace. "What do you mean," you say? By whose power do you live? Who gives you the power to talk and move and do whatever you do? It is God. So, by whose power do you sin? It is God's power. If He ceased to give you power, you would die. So, any time someone rapes someone else, they do so by whose power? God's. Any time someone kills someone else, they do so by whose power? God's. Any time someone hurts someone else, they do so by whose power? God's. Is God happy about it? No!

He tells us in Isaiah 43:24, "But thou hast made me to serve with thy sins, thou hast wearied me with thine iniquities." God has pledged Himself to maintain the life and power of we who sin, so that He may give us an opportunity to see His love and surrender our lives to Him and be saved for eternity. But while He is maintaining our life, we are causing Him to serve with our sins. God hates sin. He absolutely hates sin, because it counterworks everything that He stands for. But it is by His grace that we sin.

Free Moral Agents

You see, we are free moral agents. God loves us supremely. And He created us with the capacity to love Him in return. But love cannot be love if it is involuntary. It must be voluntary in order to be love. Love necessitates freedom of choice. And freedom of choice— of will—allows for the possibility of service, or the possibility of rebellion. In order to preserve the capacity to love, God must also preserve the capacity to be selfish, to hurt, to destroy.

What Does Love Look Like?

If love is so necessary to maintain at such extreme costs, what does love look like? Let us go to the Bible and read from the "love chapter," 1 Corinthians 13. I want to begin in verse 4, giving you my paraphrase of the text.

"Love suffers long and is kind...."[243] When I live by love all of the following will be true. I will not be exempt from suffering. In fact, I can suffer, and I can suffer for a long time. Not only that, but I can suffer for a long time and be kind while I suffer. With love, I can suffer long and be kind to the one causing my suffering.

"...love does not envy...."[244] I do not want what you have, because I recognize that God is my source, not you. I am happy that you have

---

[243] 1 Corinthians 13:4
[244] Ibid.

what you have, because the Lord has blessed you with it. I don't need your stuff. I need God.

"...love does not parade itself...."[245] I don't do things to make people look at me, notice me, or think good of me. In fact, I avoid doing things publicly that would draw attention to myself. My motivation for what I do is not what you think. It is what God thinks, and He knows the heart, so I don't need to prove anything to Him.

"is not puffed up...."[246] I don't put others down so that I feel bigger or more important. I don't try to look more holy, nicer, prettier, or anything else. I don't need fancy clothes, makeup, jewelry, a nice car, a nice home, or anything else to embellish who I am. I am content with how God has made me.

"...does not behave rudely...."[247] I do not behave rudely to those who are rude to me. I treat them with patience, kindness, compassion, and love.

"...does not seek its own...."[248] I do not seek my own rights. I will allow myself to be taken advantage of without retaliation or resistance (recognizing that if God allows it, He will work it out for good and will give me strength to endure), and I will allow God to work it out in His time and in His way. "Vengeance is mine; I will repay, saith the Lord."[249] While I do not seek my own rights, I do uphold the rights of others.

"...is not provoked...."[250] I cannot be provoked. In other words, I have no buttons. You know what I mean, right? There are some people that can easily "push our buttons." Usually those who are closest to us can push our buttons the best—like family. They know exactly what to do or say or how to say it to get us upset, frustrated, angry, etc. so that we respond in a negative way to them. It is a form of control, and because we are one of their sources, they must try to control us.

---

[245] Ibid.
[246] Ibid.
[247] 1 Corinthians 13:5
[248] Ibid.
[249] Romans 12:19
[250] 1 Corinthians 13:5

Buttons represent emotional hurts that have not been healed. Let me illustrate. You have just broken your arm in an accident, and you go to the emergency department. They take x-rays, put your arm in a sling, and send you home to follow up with the orthopedic surgeon tomorrow to have a cast put on your arm. But, while you are going home, you remember that you MUST pick up an item at the store now. In the store, someone bumps into your broken arm, and you yell at them, "Watch out! Don't be so clumsy!" They don't have a clue that your arm is broken. They might be thinking, "Why are you so grumpy!?"

Your response to them bumping into you is not because of what they did, it is because of how you feel. If you didn't have a broken arm, you might not even have noticed that they bumped into you, or if you did, it wouldn't be a big deal. The bigger the hurt, the more easily a response is evoked and the more exaggerated the response is. Also, the more unhealed hurts that there are, the more buttons there are to "push."

If you are someone who is always responding negatively to others, and you don't know why, it is probably because you have suffered many hurts which have not healed yet. You need a personal experience at the foot of the cross where Jesus can take your hurts and give you His hurt-free life in exchange. Love has no buttons, because love heals all the hurts from the past. And when you have no buttons, you cannot be provoked.

When someone responds poorly to you, remember they aren't responding to you, per se. They are responding to their internal pain. Be gentle and patient with them. They are still hurting.

"...thinks no evil...."[251] I think no evil about you. I assume that your motives are pure for why you are doing what you do. I understand where you are coming from, and in compassion I pray for you, work with you, and am patient with you. My thoughts about you are always positive.

---

[251] Ibid.

"...does not rejoice in iniquity, but rejoices in the truth...."[252] It gives me no pleasure when you sin, fall, or fail. My concern is for your best good. Your sin hurts me, because I hurt for you and what that sin is doing in your life. I cry for you in prayer, interceding on your behalf and lifting you up before My Father in heaven. And it is my greatest joy and rejoicing when you receive the truth in your life and the truth sets you free.

"...bears all things...."[253] Love is able to carry anything, no matter how big or how bad. There is nothing—in my life, in my associations, in my experience—that God is not acquainted with and has not made provision for. God, who is love, can and did bear it all. And knowing me intimately, He has pledged that He will not allow anything to come to me that I cannot bear. Therefore, I can bear all things that come to me, because they are filtered by God first so that not one of them is too great. By His grace, I can overcome in each and every situation and temptation. Love leaves me no excuses for failure, because it gives me everything needed to overcome.

"...believes all things...."[254] Love believes all things that God has promised, because I know who He is and how trustworthy He is and have proved Him by personal experience many times in the past, and my faith has grown to the point that I happily surrender all to Him.

"...hopes all things...."[255] Love has great hope, because I know that God is trustworthy, and I can confidently hope for what He has promised.

"...endures all things...."[256] Love is able to withstand anything and everything. Love is the greatest power in existence—there is no greater power. Force, coercion, shame, guilt, threats, abuse, deception, temptation—are all powerless to overcome love, because it is infinitely greater than all these things. There will never be anything that can

---

[252] 1 Corinthians 13:6
[253] 1 Corinthians 13:7
[254] Ibid.
[255] Ibid.
[256] Ibid.

wear me down and outdo my endurance if love is the motivation and experience of my life. I will endure to the end, only by love.

"...love never fails."[257] Because of what love is and Who love is, it will not—cannot—fail. It will be victorious at last!

Now, let us go back to the first part of 1 Corinthians 13 and read more about this love. "Though I speak with the tongues of men and of angels, but have not [this] love, I have become sounding brass or a clanging cymbal. And though I have the gift of prophecy, and understand all mysteries and all knowledge, and though I have all faith, so that I could remove mountains, but have not [this] love, I am nothing. And though I bestow all my goods to feed the poor, and though I give my body to be burned, but have not [this] love, it profits me nothing."

John 7:21-23 states the following, "Not everyone who says to Me, 'Lord, Lord,' shall enter the kingdom of heaven, but he who does the will of My Father in heaven. Many will say to Me in that day, 'Lord, Lord, have we not prophesied in Your name, cast out demons in Your name, and done many wonders in Your name?' And then I will declare to them, 'I never knew you; depart from Me, you who practice lawlessness!'" What we have read in 1 Corinthians 13 and here is John 7:21-23 tells me this: selfishness can do so much "apparent" good that it fools many into believing it is the real thing (even the one who is doing it), when God knows that it is not.

How can God say, "I never knew you," to those who were apparently working for Him? It is because there is one thing that God recognizes—love. And if there is no love in you and me—if we are operating from the old heart of selfishness and pride—He doesn't recognize us.

Does God recognize you? If not, you must come to and stay at the cross, pleading for the new heart, until you are assured that you have it. Then plead for Him to live out His life in you through the Holy Spirit, to keep you in that new heart.

---

[257] 1 Corinthians 13:8

CHAPTER FIFTEEN

A Love that Heals

8. Remember, It's Not Mine

I need to remember—it's not mine! This is a frequent challenge. We have been so accustomed to treating things and people and relationships as if they are ours, when they actually belong to God. We frequently find ourselves in the situation where we are treating something or someone like it is ours—like it belongs to us—and we need to be reminded that it isn't ours, and to surrender the control of all things to God who does own it, so that He can work things out in His way. I simply need to trust Him in each and every situation that He will work out the best for me. I don't need to take things personally. I can be just like the UPS delivery guy, unhurt by what others say and do, because it's not about me. It's not mine!

For example, my struggle frequently revolves around certain children not obeying or respecting their mother and father. When I get frustrated, it is because I have forgotten that It's not mine. I am frustrated because I see them as my children, and I believe they are defying my (or my wife's) authority. It is in times like this that I need to pause for a moment and remember, it's not mine! Yes, Lord. They are Your children. And any authority I have has only been delegated by You, so it is Your authority. So, Lord, how would You have me respond to Your children using Your authority?

When I gain this perspective, I no longer have the frustration and anxiety as before, because I am only a steward of His resources, not the owner. I am not the one offended, so I don't have to act offended. It is a liberating experience. But, I frequently forget this truth, so I must frequently remember it again.

Love, Trust, and Protection

Now, let us consider love, trust, and protection. If I love God, I can trust Him, correct? And If I trust in God, do I need to protect myself? No, I can trust in Him to protect me as He sees fit.

In Luke 6:27-36 we read, "Love your enemies, do good to those who hate you, bless those who curse you, and pray for those who spitefully use you."[258] The old heart cannot do this. It is only the new heart, recreated by the love and grace of God, that can respond with love to those who hate you, curse you, and spitefully use you. Don't be mistaken, thinking that when you have love you will be loved by all.

Love—real love—is hated by many. Many will consider you their enemy. But you will not consider any of them as your enemy.

"To him who strikes you on the one cheek..."[259] strike him back? Give him a good karate chop? Defend yourself? The natural response is to defend oneself, to not allow oneself to be taken advantage of. It is only by the strength of God that I can allow someone to take advantage of me, and then to allow them to take advantage of me again. Why would I do that? God surrounds me with His presence, and nothing can get through to harm me, unless He gives permission. So, if someone punches me in the face, the only

[258] Luke 6:27,28
[259] Luke 6:29

way they can do it is if God allows it. And if God allows it, it is because He will work it out for good, and He will give me strength to endure.

I don't have to protect myself. I don't have to fear evil. I can trust in God to care for me, because He knows what is best. "To him who strikes you on the one cheek, offer the other also."[260]

"And from him who takes away your [house], do not withhold your [car] either."[261] A common scenario that I meet in my practice is bitterness over a divorce. The relationship has gone south, and both are at loss, so a divorce is filed. One wants to get as much as they can, to the detriment of the other. If you are in that situation, what does this text say to you? If your soon-to-be ex-spouse takes you to divorce court and takes the house away from you, give them the car also. In the first case, you are a victim. In the second, you are a donor. We are blessed by giving, not by losing. So, turn your loss into a gift, and you win more than good health.

"And from him who takes away your goods do not ask them back."[262] If you are taken to court and sued, even if it is wrongly, don't go back and counter sue. Let them have it. It wasn't yours anyway. It was God's. And If He lets them have it, He can give you more when He knows the right time and circumstances are in place. Just trust yourself in God's care. Paul tells us, "Beloved, do not avenge yourselves, but rather give place to wrath; for it is written, 'Vengeance is Mine, I will repay,' says the Lord. Therefore 'If your enemy is hungry, feed him; if he is thirsty, give him a drink; for in so doing you will heap coals of fire on his head.' Do not be overcome by evil, but overcome evil with good."[263]

"And just as you want men to do to you, you also do to them likewise."[264] This "Golden Rule" will be our every-day rule, when love rules in our hearts. We will be concerned about the other, not ourselves.

---

[260] Ibid.
[261] Ibid.
[262] Luke 6:30
[263] Romans 12:19-21
[264] Luke 6:31

We will do whatever we can to show them the love of God. Our yearning will be for them and their salvation, even if they are treating us terribly. This is the way love is.

"But if you love those who love you, what credit is that to you? For even sinners love those who love them. And if you do good to those who do good to you, what credit is that to you? For even sinners do the same. And if you lend to those from whom you hope to receive back, what credit is that to you? For even sinners lend to sinners to receive as much back."[265] Selfishness can mimic love—part of the time. But only love can be love all of the time. Selfishness can "love." It can "do good." It can lend cheerfully. But the motives are entirely different than true love.

"But love your enemies, do good, and lend, hoping for nothing in return; and your reward will be great, and you will be sons of the Most High. For He is kind to the unthankful and evil. Therefore be merciful, just as your Father also is merciful."[266] That is the God we serve. He is love. And this is how love acts. What an awesome God we serve! I want to be like Him!

This is love, friends—real love. And it is impossible for us to generate this kind of love. Real love is divine, and I can only possess this love if Christ lives in my heart by faith.

"...it is only the Spirit of God that gives love for hatred. To be kind to the unthankful and to the evil, to do good hoping for nothing again, is the insignia of the royalty of heaven, the sure token by which the children of the Highest reveal their high estate."[267] Do you want to know if you are really a child of God? The possession of love guarantees it!

---

[265] Luke 6:32-34
[266] Luke 6:35,36
[267] White, E. G. (1896) *Thoughts from the Mount of Blessing.* (p 75). Mountain View, CA: Pacific Press Publishing Association.

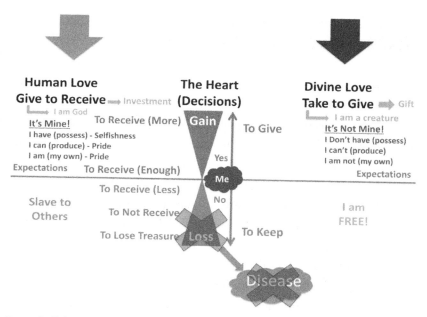

Love & Disease

Now that we have covered the topic of love more adequately, let us consider disease again. The Ministry of Healing, page 127, beautifully describes how we should understand and approach sickness. It says, "Disease is an effort of nature to free the system from conditions that result from a violation of the laws of health."[268] This tells me that disease is a good thing—it is the "effort of nature to free the system..." It is good to have my system free, so disease is on the good side of the equation. It is not disease that is bad, it is the violation of the laws of health that is bad. When the laws of health are violated, it causes conditions which the body tries to free itself from, and the effort of freeing itself from those conditions is called disease.

Next, we are told, "In the case of sickness, the cause should be ascertained."[269] So, when there is a case of sickness or disease, our first work is to find the cause. We have already learned that 90% of

---

[268] White, E. G. (1905) *The Ministry of Healing.* (p 127). Mountain View, CA: Pacific Press Publishing Association.
[269] Ibid.

diseases have their foundation in the mind. And of those mind issues, personal loss is a large cause of disease.

If I live under the old heart of human love, giving to receive, I am constantly living in personal loss, because I didn't receive, I didn't receive enough, or my treasures were taken away. I can't control those losses, because I am dependent upon others to give or receive and I cannot control if someone rejects me or dies. That accumulated loss leads to physical disease over time. And the greater the perceived loss, the more rapid and serious the physical decline.

But if I live by God's heart, operating with divine love, which is taking to give, then my only loss is if I keep His love to myself. Otherwise, I am not at loss, and all of those things which had contributed to my physical degeneration no longer do so, for they are no longer part of the equation. So, if there is no more loss in the new heart, then there is no more contribution to disease from that source. And if the cause is removed...the effect must cease!

Which Heart Do I Have?

So, if my personal losses have so much to do with my physical health, and if my losses are dependent upon which heart I have, how do I know which heart I have? There are several things that differentiate the old heart from the new one.

The old heart gives to receive, while the new heart takes to give.

The old heart *invests* in others, while the new heart *gives* to others. The old heart wins or gains by receiving from others, while the new heart wins or gains by giving. The old heart is at loss when it doesn't receive, when it doesn't receive enough, or when its treasure is taken away, while the new heart is only at loss if it keeps to itself that which it took from God.

The old heart believes that it's mine, while the new heart believes that it's *NOT* mine. The old heart believes that I possess it, while the new heart believes that I *DON'T* possess it. The old heart believes that I can produce it, while the new heart believes that I *CAN'T* produce it. The old heart believes that I am my own, while the old heart believes that I am *NOT* my own.

The old heart gets impatient and angry when someone does it wrong, while the new heart suffers long under persecution and is kind while it suffers. The old heart wants what others have, while the new heart does not envy. The old heart does things to be noticed by others, while the new heart does not parade itself and its supposed goodness. The old heart tries to make itself look better than it really is, while the new heart is not puffed up, recognizing that its goodness is only in Christ, not itself.

The old heart is rude to those who are rude to it, while the new heart doesn't behave rudely to anyone, regardless of how they treat it.

The old heart always tries to protect its own rights, while the new heart does not seek its own rights. Rather, it seeks the rights of others.

The old heart gets angry or frustrated when others do it wrong, while the new heart cannot be provoked. The old heart surmises or suspects evil of others, while the new heart thinks no evil of others. It assumes that others are doing what they are doing from the best of motives.

The old heart is happy when its enemies fall, because that makes self look better, while the new heart does not rejoice in iniquity or others sins or faults. The old heart likes to hear and participate in rumors and gossip, while the new heart rejoices in the truth and rejoices when the truth sets others free.

The old heart can't stand it when _____ (you fill in the blank), while the new heart bears all things that come its way. The old heart just can't believe _____ (you fill in the blank), while the new heart believes all things God has said, regardless of what things you face.

The old heart feels hopeless about certain things from time to time, while the new heart hopes all things that have been promised.

The old heart is easily overcome by temptation and trial, while the new heart endures all things that happen to it. The old heart loves those who love it and are nice to it. The new heart also loves...but it loves its enemies. The old heart does good to those who are good to it. The new heart also does good...but it does good to those that hate it. The old heart blesses those that bless it. The new heart also blesses...but it blesses those who curse it. The old heart prays for those who are kind to it and are loved by it. The new heart also prays...but it prays for those who spitefully use it and mistreat it.

The old heart turns and retaliates when it is attacked. The new heart also turns...but it turns the other cheek when taken advantage of. The old heart gives only what is demanded of it. The new heart also gives...but it gives more than is demanded. The old heart gives occasionally when asked. The new heart also gives...but it gives every time when asked and when the fulfillment of the request would be for good.

The old heart asks back everything that was wrongfully taken from it, and sometimes it asks for more. The new heart also asks back...but it asks back nothing that was wrongfully taken from it. The old heart does to others as it believes they deserve. The new heart also does to others...but the new heart does to others as it would have them to do it.

The old heart gives hoping for them to give back so it can receive. The new heart also gives...but the new heart gives without hoping for anything in return from them. It is a gift. The old heart is personally hurt when others don't treat it well, while the new heart is *NOT* personally hurt when others don't treat it well. The old heart is motivated by selfishness, while the new heart is motivated by love.

Love & Disease

Is disease only the result of a love problem? Of personal loss? No! But 90% of it is! Remember, we are told, "Sickness of the mind prevails everywhere. Nine tenths of the diseases from which men suffer have their foundation here."[270] So, if 90% of our illnesses have their foundation in the mind, and a lack of divine love is the source of those mind issues, then it makes sense to search for a cause for one's disease or illness here first.

But not only do we seek for the cause, The Ministry of Healing, p. 127 goes on to say, "Unhealthful conditions should be changed..."[271] Not only are we to identify the cause of the disease, but we need to adopt a healthy lifestyle.

---

[270] White, E. G. (1923) *Counsels on Health.* (p 324). Mountain View, CA: Pacific Press Publishing Association.
[271] White, E. G. (1905) *The Ministry of Healing.* (p 127). Mountain View, CA: Pacific Press Publishing Association.

CHAPTER SIXTEEN

A Love that Obeys

9. Use Natural Remedies, Change My Lifestyle

Y ou and I, in response to God's love for us, should use the means that God has placed in our pathway to improve the health of our bodies. This includes using natural remedies and changing our lifestyle.

In doing so, we STAND for WELLNESS. Wellness stands for **W**ater, **E**xercise, **L**ive Temperately, **L**ove, **N**utrition, **E**nvironment, which includes **S**unshine, our **T**hought life, **A**ir, **N**ature, and **D**ress. Wellness also includes **S**ufficient rest and **S**imple trust in God. So, we STAND for WELLNESS!

The Ministry of Healing, p. 127 goes on to explain that, "wrong habits [should be] corrected."[272] We have wrong habits of dressing. We have wrong habits of thinking. We have wrong habits of eating. We have wrong habits of drinking. And these habits need to be corrected. We need to develop right habits, one choice at a time.

---

[272] White, E. G. (1905) *The Ministry of Healing.* (p 127). Mountain View, CA: Pacific Press Publishing Association.

Finally, The Ministry of Healing, p. 127 states, "Then nature is to be assisted in her effort to expel impurities and to re-establish right conditions in the system."[273] We use hydrotherapy, herbs, good food, exercise, and other simple, natural remedies to assist in the healing process. We attempt to expel impurities, and we work at re-establishing the right conditions, opposition to the wrong conditions that were the result of violating the laws of health. In the case of sickness, we do all of this.

And the Bible gives us another method that we can follow in the case of sickness. This is outlined in James chapter 5, verses 14 through 16. "Is anyone among you sick? Let him call for the elders of the church, and let them pray over him, anointing him with oil in the name of the Lord. And the prayer of faith will save the sick, and the Lord will raise him up. And if he has committed sins, he will be forgiven. Confess your trespasses to one another, and pray for one another, that you may be healed. The effective, fervent prayer of a righteous man avails much." Do not overlook this scriptural admonition in the case of sickness.

Disease & Lifestyle

Why do I adopt a healthy lifestyle? God loves me, and He purchased me at an infinite price. I love Him, because He first loved me. And I take care of my body in proportion to the price He paid for it. I live as healthy as possible in order to preserve my body in the best condition possible, because my body is His temple.

We are reminded of this in 1 Corinthians 6:19,20, "Or do you not know that your body is the temple of the Holy Spirit who is in you, whom you have from God, and you are not your own? For you were bought at a price; therefore glorify God in your body and in your spirit, which are God's."

---

[273] White, E. G. (1905) *The Ministry of Healing*. (p 127). Mountain View, CA: Pacific Press Publishing Association.

But why do I obey? Why am I looking for healing? What is my motive? Why I do what I do is at least as important as what I do. Do I obey in order to be healed? No! That is operating under the system of human love, giving to receive. I obey because I love God, and I want to give him the gift of service, in gratitude for what He has done for me. The latter response is living by divine love, which is taking to give.

When I take of God's love, it transforms me. The desire of my heart, which is influenced by that love, is to obey the one I love. And that obedience includes taking care of my body for Christ. Jesus tells us, "If you love Me, keep My commandments."[274] And He reminds us, "He who has My commandments and keeps them, it is he who loves Me."[275] True obedience is the fruit of love.

Cause & Effect

Again, we are reminded of the law of cause and effect. My disease must have a cause. The cause always comes before the disease develops. As long as the disease is present, the cause or its secondary causes are still present. If the cause is a love or sin issues, I can change my lifestyle or take my medications, but if I don't remove the love or sin issue, some other manifestation will come from that cause, and I will be worse off than when I started.

Yes, we are to adopt healthy lifestyles. Yes, we are to use simple, natural remedies. But most importantly, the cause must be identified and removed, because once the cause is removed, the effect will cease. But in the meantime, I apply the lifestyle principles, I use the natural remedies, and I eliminate the toxins through various natural treatments.

We can reason from cause to effect because there is a law that governs cause and effect.

---

[274] John 14:15
[275] John 14:21

Law of Function

We see that all laws that govern function are unchangeable. The laws of thermodynamics are unchangeable. The law of gravity is unchangeable. The law of body temperature, which governs what temperature range our bodies function at optimally, is unchangeable. I can't just decide that I don't like these laws and that they won't apply to my life. I can't just decide to act outside of the laws of thermodynamics or of gravity, or that I will live just fine with a body temperature of negative 30 degrees. It matters not how much I like or don't like these laws or how much I want to abide by them or not. They are the laws that govern these functions.

So, what about the Law of Life? What about God's law? Is it just a moral law, or is it a law of function? It is a law of function. It is the law which governs the function of love.

I can't just decide I don't like it. I can't just decide that I will change it. I can't just decide that I won't abide by it or that it doesn't apply to me. No, the law is a functional law, and it cannot be changed. And if I break this law, whether deliberately or ignorantly, there will be consequences. But if I keep this law, by God's grace and with the heart that He gives me, there will be consequences as well—consequences of life, love, peace, and joy.

What do the commandments say? "I am the Lord your God, who brought you out of the land of Egypt, out of the house of bondage.

You shall have no other gods before Me. You shall not make for yourself a carved image—any likeness of anything that is in heaven above, or that is in the earth beneath, or that is in the water under the earth; you shall not bow down to them nor serve them. For I, the Lord your God, am a jealous God, visiting the iniquity of the fathers upon the children to the third and fourth generations of those who hate Me, but showing mercy to thousands, to those who love Me and keep My commandments. You shall not take the name of the Lord your God in vain, for the Lord will not hold him guiltless who takes His name in vain.

Remember the Sabbath day, to keep it holy. Six days you shall labor and do all your work, but the seventh day is the Sabbath of the Lord your God. In it you shall do no work: you, nor your son, nor your daughter, nor your male servant, nor your female servant, nor your cattle, nor your stranger who is within your gates. For in six days the Lord made the heavens and the earth, the sea, and all that is in them, and rested the seventh day. Therefore the Lord blessed the Sabbath day and hallowed it.

Honor your father and your mother, that your days may be long upon the land which the Lord your God is giving you. You shall not murder. You shall not commit adultery. You shall not steal. You shall not bear false witness against your neighbor. You shall not covet your neighbor's house; you shall not covet your neighbor's wife, nor his male servant, nor his female servant, nor his ox, nor his donkey, nor anything that is your neighbor's."[276]

This is the law that governs the function of love—the taking love and the giving love. It is the law the reveals to us how love functions and shows how everything is to be ordered according to the character and likeness of God.

What is the relationship between Jesus and the law? Did Jesus come to the earth to do away with the law? No! He says, "Do not think that I came to destroy the Law or the Prophets. I did not come to destroy but to fulfill. For assuredly, I say to you, till heaven and earth pass away, one jot or one tittle will by no means pass from the law till all is fulfilled."[277] Jesus didn't come to destroy the law. He came to fulfill it.

But what did He come to fulfill? If you break the law and run a red light and hit another car, causing damage to that other car, is there a penalty for breaking the law? Yes, there is. There is a

---

[276] Exodus 20:2-17
[277] Matthew 5:17,18

penalty—a fine—that is attached to the breaking of the law. And someone must pay for the damage that was done to the other car. Who has to pay? The one who broke the law and caused the accident.

You and I, from Adam and Eve on down, have broken the law, which is sin ("For all have sinned and fall short of the glory of God."[278] "Whosoever committeth sin transgresseth also the law: for sin is the transgression of the law."[279]), and the penalty for breaking the law is death ("For the wages of sin *is* death."[280]).

Jesus came, as we have already discussed, to live a perfect life in human flesh to be able to provide for us a perfect past (which the law requires). But He also came to pay for us the penalty of the broken law and the damage that the breaking of that law caused.

If God could have changed the law, then Jesus did not need to come to pay its penalty. The law could simply be changed to meet the circumstances, and Jesus would not have had to come and be tortured to death. But the fact that Jesus did come and suffer and die shows us that the law could not be changed. It is, remember, the law of love—the law that reveals what the character of God is like and how it is to be reflected in the life of His creatures.

But the law was nailed to the cross, wasn't it? Paul says, "And you, being dead in your trespasses and the uncircumcision of your flesh, He has made alive together with Him, having forgiven you all trespasses, having wiped out the handwriting of requirements that was against us, which was contrary to us. And He has taken it out of the way, having nailed it to the cross."[281] What here is nailed to the cross? It is "the handwriting of requirements that was against us." What is Paul referring to? Is he referring to the law of God which reveals to us the character—the love—of God, the law that governs the function of love?

---

[278] Romans 3:23
[279] 1 John 3:4 KJV
[280] Romans 6:23
[281] Colossians 2:13,14

We find what Paul is referring to in Deuteronomy 31:24-26, where it says, "So it was, when Moses had completed writing the words of this law in a book, when they were finished, that Moses commanded the Levites, who bore the ark of the covenant of the Lord, saying: 'Take this Book of the Law, and put it beside the ark of the covenant of the Lord your God, that it may be there as a witness against you.'" Here is a document which contained the handwriting of Moses which was specifically placed beside the ark "as a witness against you." What was Moses writing about? It was not the 10 commandments, the law of God, the law of love. He was writing about the ordinances or covenants with the associated curses for disobeying God.

The ten commandments were placed *inside* the ark of the covenant, not beside it. "He took the Testimony and put it into the ark, inserted the poles through the rings of the ark, and put the mercy seat on top of the ark."[282] "Nothing was in the ark except the two tablets of stone which Moses put there at Horeb, when the Lord made a covenant with the children of Israel, when they came out of the land of Egypt."[283]

Paul expands upon this thought, "having abolished in His [Jesus'] flesh the enmity, that is, the law of commandments contained in ordinances, so as to create in Himself one new man from the two [Jew & Gentile, circumcised & uncircumcised], thus making peace, and that He might reconcile them both to God in one body through the cross, thereby putting to death the enmity."[284]

We see here that what was nailed to the cross in the person of Jesus was not the law of God, which is the law of love, but rather the ordinances of the ceremonial law which pointed forward to the coming Messiah and the sacrifice He would make. When Jesus lived a perfect life (the Lamb without spot or blemish) and died for our sin,

---

[282] Exodus 40:20
[283] 1 Kings 8:9
[284] Ephesians 2:15,16

The Law of Life

He in reality fulfilled what the sacrificial system pointed to in symbol. That sacrificial system could no longer function to point people forward, by faith, to the sacrifice that the Messiah would make for their sin, because that sacrifice was already made. It was, therefore, nailed to the cross. The law of God—the law of love—however, could not be changed. It is a functional law.

Is there anyone here who has ever sinned? All of us? What is the definition of sin? It is the transgression of the law. If sin is the transgression of the law and you still sin, there must still be a law to transgress. Other translations say that sin is lawlessness. That is, sin is living or acting as if there is no law. It is living or acting without regard to the law. It is like speeding when there are clearly defined speed limits, running red lights or stop signs, and parking in handicapped spaces when you are not handicapped.

Did the life and death of Jesus somehow make it okay to have other gods before God? Did His life and death make it okay to worship idols/images? Did it make it okay to take God's name in vain? What about to dishonor your parents, murder others, commit adultery, steal, lie, and covet? Are all of those things all of a sudden okay because they were nailed to the cross with Jesus? No! That's ridiculous! The whole Christian world can see that these commands are still binding. But what about the one commandment that bids us remember, as if God knew we would forget?

"Remember the Sabbath day, to keep it holy. Six days you shall labor and do all your work, but the seventh day is the Sabbath of the Lord your God. In it you shall do no work: you, nor your son, nor your daughter, nor your male servant, nor your female servant, nor your cattle, nor your stranger who is within your gates. For in six days the Lord made the heavens and the earth, the sea, and all that is in them, and rested the seventh day. Therefore the Lord blessed the Sabbath day and hallowed it."[285]

---

[285] Exodus 20:8-11

262

The Law of Life

Does it matter to God what day is set aside for His worship? Does it matter to the groom which woman he marries? There is the bride and six bridesmaids. Why doesn't he just choose one of the bridesmaids and marry her and not the bride? Would it matter? Yes, it would matter! There are seven days in the week. Does it make a difference to God which day He has set apart? The day that God has chosen is important to Him, and it should be important to us.

Even at creation, God knew what was best for us, and in knowing what was best for us, He gave us the Sabbath—the seventh-day Sabbath. "And on the seventh day God ended His work which He had done, and He rested on the seventh day from all His work which He had done. Then God blessed the seventh day and sanctified it, because in it He rested from all His work which God had created and made."[286] For more information on the topic, please visit www.sabbathtruth.com.

So, what If I keep nine of the ten commandments? Isn't that good enough? James makes it clear to us, "For whoever shall keep the whole law, and yet stumble in one point, he is guilty of all."[287] This means that if you and I are keeping nine of the ten commandments, but you are breaking one, you are still a law breaker, you are still living your own way regardless of the law, you are still sinning against God and His law.

Remember, sin is breaking the law—God's law, which has love as its foundation. And in many cases, disease is the result of a love problem. The world is sick because of sin, and it is our privilege to come to God, to be empowered by His Holy Spirit, that in us, Christ may overcome sin and set us free by His love. "Behold! The Lamb of God who takes away the sin of the world!"[288]

---

[286] Genesis 2:2,3
[287] James 2:10
[288] John 1:29

CHAPTER SEVENTEEN

A Love that Overcomes

10. Get (Back) Up

Our tenth and final point is to get up or get back up. To begin illustrating this point, let us go to John 5:2-8 and consider the story of the lame man by the pool of Bethesda. "Now there is in Jerusalem by the Sheep Gate a pool, which is called in Hebrew, Bethesda, having five porches. In these lay a great multitude of sick people, blind, lame, paralyzed...Now a certain man was there who had an infirmity thirty-eight years. When Jesus saw him lying there, and knew that he already had been in that condition a long time, He said to him, 'Do you want to be made well?'...Jesus said to him, 'Rise, take up your bed and walk.' And immediately the man was made well, took up his bed, and walked."

Let us analyze, step by step, what happened in the healing of this man, because this act of healing is an example of how God wants to make us successful.

First of all, Jesus gave the man a command—to take up his bed and walk. There was definite instruction that was given to the man. He was made aware of what he was expected to do.

In order to take Jesus' word, the man had to put his trust in Jesus. He had to believe in Him and what He said. He had to exercise faith in Jesus and His word.

The Bible tells us that faith works. So, when this man exercised his faith in Jesus, he then acted upon that faith to attempt to accomplish what Jesus had commanded him to do, even though he had no capacity in himself to accomplish the task.

Once the man believed in Jesus and initiated the attempt to comply with the command, he was given Divine power to actually be able to accomplish what the command specified. But it was only after faith acted upon the command that he was given the power to accomplish it. And, finally, the man was healed in the process of acting, by faith, upon the command of Jesus.

As we ponder this sequence of events, we discover why many of us have led unsuccessful lives, even in the spiritual realm. We have listened to lies ever since we were born, and we are used to believing these lies. So, when Jesus comes along and gives us a command that goes against these lies, we don't trust Him. We don't believe that it is possible to accomplish what He is asking of us. And if we don't believe, if we don't trust Him, if we don't exercise faith in His word, we will never overcome. I pray that the rest of what we have covered together in the Law of Life convinces you that you can and must trust God, and not yourself, not your feelings, not other's opinions, etc.

Another problem is that we want evidence of the power or healing before we act upon the command. When Jesus told the man to get up, if the man would have said, "Lord, make me well, and I will get up," what do you think would have happened? He wouldn't have been healed. He had to act by faith upon the command itself, and when he did so, the power and healing came. It is the same with us. If we wait until we feel strong enough or feel healed and whole before we begin to trust in and act upon God's commands and promises, we never will act upon them. And if we never act upon them, they will never do us any good. We will remain sick, powerless, and defeated. So, getting up is an act of faith, responding to the command or promise of God, making the effort to accomplish what was commanded or promised, and being empowered by God in the very act to be able to accomplish what was commanded or promised.

Learning to Walk

So how do we understand falling down? Let's say that you have, by faith, gotten up from your sinful state and have stood for the right. But soon after that, you fall back down. What do you do? Many of us, myself included, have been in the habit of wining, fussing, throwing an adult temper tantrum, staying on the ground and refusing to get back up. But how does a baby learn how to walk?

Babies are very uncoordinated. About the age of 9 or 10 months of age, they begin to pull themselves up into a standing position next to furniture or other stable objects. Then as time progresses, they learn to scoot along, holding on to the furniture. But one day, they let go and look across the room at some desired object, and something momentous happens. They take a step! And what happens right after they take a step? They fall!

And how do the parents respond? The parents are excited that their baby took its first step! Do they get angry at their baby and spank them and tell them how horrible they are because they fell? No, that is ridiculous. The parents know that the baby will fall—many times—in the process of learning how to walk. They are just excited that their baby is taking its first steps and learning how to walk!

But most of the time we think of God as an angry God. We believe He is watching for every opportunity to find fault in us so that

He can condemn us. We believe that every time we fall, He is angry and disappointed with us. But that is not the case at all.

He is the Good Shepherd in search of the lost sheep. He is the woman sweeping the home for the lost coin. He is the father scanning the horizon every day, watching for the return of His prodigal child. And He knows that learning to walk always involves falling—always. It is not a problem for God that we fall. He already paid the price for each fall on the cross. He already suffered the penalty for each sin. He already knew that each fall was going to come before it ever did, and He made provision for it.

We are told that "a righteous man may fall seven times and rise again."[289] Notice a couple things. It is a righteous man that falls. He falls multiple times. But in order to fall more than once, you have to get up and then fall again. So, a righteous man gets up, falls down, and gets back up again. The problem is not falling down. The problem is not getting back up.

You see, many times when we fall, we refuse to get back up again. It's like we have a temper tantrum when we fall. We listen to the lies of the enemy telling us that we should "just give up. It doesn't work anyway. You always were a failure and you always will be. You can't even go to God now, because you messed up and He won't hear you. Just face it, you'll never make it." So, we believe the lies and we sit on the ground, unwilling and unable to get back up.

But God is there, trying to encourage you to get back up. Just as when He spoke to the man by the pool of Bethesda, Jesus speaks to you and me, saying, "Get back up." And just like that man, we have a choice. We can either trust in Jesus and His command/promise, act upon that command, and be empowered to be able to accomplish the task, or we can trust the lies, distrust Jesus, and fail to act upon his command/promise. If latter is our response, we will always stay on the ground, unable to get back up, like that man was for 38 years. But

---

[289] Proverbs 24:16

when we trust Jesus and believe His word, when we act upon His command, He empowers us to be able to accomplish that which He commands. A righteous man falls seven times and gets back up and keeps going. And I suspect it isn't just seven times.

Jesus tells us, "I do not say to you, up to seven times, but up to seventy times seven."[290] How many times will you allow your child to fall in the process of learning to walk? Would you cut it off at 7 times? How about 490 times? I suspect neither. You would allow them as many times to fall as is necessary for them to learn to walk. The same is true of God. He will allow you as many times as it takes. So, stop beating yourself up. It doesn't help you to do so.

Believe that God loves you. Believe that He has your best interests in mind. Believe that He is better to you than earthly parents ever could be. Believe that He has already forgiven your sin and made provision for you to get back up. Believe that He offers you, right now in the midst of your fall, the power to get back up and keep moving on toward victory.

Keep in mind that God's grace and forgiveness is not a license for sin. "What shall we say then? Shall we continue in sin that grace may abound? Certainly not! How shall we who died to sin live any longer in it?"[291]

God's grace is not there to make us unconcerned about falling and staying on the ground. It is not there to make us feel that we can just fall any time we purposely want to, and it's okay. When we see how much God loves us, when we see the sacrifice that He made for us on the cross, when we see how much of a treasure God is and how valuable we are to him, when we see that every sin wounds the heart of God and added to the pain that Jesus bore on the cross, when we see that sin separates us from the very One who loves us so much and the very One we love in return, then we constantly move away from

---

[290] Matthew 18:22
[291] Romans 6:1,2

that sin toward the righteousness of Christ. We grow in Christ so that we walk more and fall less.

Just like a child learning how to walk, we progress, improve, get up quicker, stay up longer, fall down less frequently, are more stable, are able to conquer more and more difficult terrain, and eventually we are able to "run and not be weary,"[292] and "walk and not faint."[293] We will be able to "mount up with wings like eagles,"[294] and we will become all that God created us to be.

In this Christian walk, you will fall. Expect it. But by His grace, you can get back up and continue the journey. Along the way, we become more and more like Jesus. And at the end of the road, there are blessings unimaginable.

"To him who overcomes I will grant to sit with Me on My throne, as I also overcame and sat down with My Father on His throne."[295] I don't know if God has ever offered any other creature the ability to sit on His throne, but He promises that if we overcome—if we, by faith, keep getting back up—He will allow us to rule all of creation along with Him when He returns to take us with Him to heaven. I want to be there, don't you?

Solution Summary

So, what is the solution to my problems?

1. Come & Take from God's love

We must come to God and take from His love. "Supreme love for God and unselfish love for one another—this is the best gift that our heavenly Father can bestow. This love is not an impulse, but a divine principle, a permanent power. The unconsecrated heart cannot originate or produce it. Only in the heart where Jesus reigns is

---

[292] Isaiah 40:31
[293] Ibid.
[294] Ibid.
[295] Revelation 3:21

it found. "We love Him, because He first loved us." In the heart renewed by divine grace, love is the ruling principle of action. It modifies the character, governs the impulses, controls the passions, and ennobles the affections. This love, cherished in the soul, sweetens the life and sheds a refining influence on all around."[296]

Taking of that divine love makes us look like this.

2. Accept A New Heart / New Love

I must accept a new heart, which brings to me a new love. This love does not give to receive, it takes to give. And taking to give sets me free.

3. Accept the Divine Exchange at the Cross

I need to come to the cross and accept by faith the divine exchange made possible for me by God's grace, accepting the free gift of Jesus' perfect past in exchange for my sinful one, experiencing the brokenness and transformation of the amazing love of God, and being set free from being the perpetrator and the victim.

4. Surrender My Life Entirely to Him

I need to surrender my life entirely to Him. I need to let go of the rope, get into the wheelbarrow, and put 100% trust in Jesus to get me across to the land of victory.

"'I am the Vine, ye are the branches,' Christ said to His disciples. Though He was about to be removed from them, their spiritual union with Him was to be unchanged. The connection of the branch with the vine, He said, represents the relation you are to sustain to Me. The scion is engrafted into the living vine, and fiber by fiber, vein by vein, it grows into the vine stock. The life of the vine becomes the life of the branch. So the soul dead in trespasses and sins receives life through connection with Christ. By faith in Him as a

---

[296] White, E. G. (1911). *The Acts of the Apostles.* (p 551). Mountain View, CA: Pacific Press Publishing Association.

personal Saviour the union is formed. The sinner unites his weakness to Christ's strength, his emptiness to Christ's fullness, his frailty to Christ's enduring might. Then he has the mind of Christ. The humanity of Christ has touched our humanity, and our humanity has touched divinity. Thus through the agency of the Holy Spirit man becomes a partaker of the divine nature. He is accepted in the Beloved. This union with Christ, once formed, must be maintained. Christ said, 'Abide in Me, and I in you. As the branch cannot bear fruit of itself, except it abide in the vine; no more can ye, except ye abide in Me.' This is no casual touch, no off-and-on connection. The branch becomes a part of the living vine. The communication of life, strength, and fruitfulness from the root to the branches is unobstructed and constant. Separated from the vine, the branch cannot live. No more, said Jesus, can you live apart from Me. The life you have received from Me can be preserved only by continual communion. Without Me you cannot overcome one sin, or resist one temptation.

'Abide in Me, and I in you.' Abiding in Christ means a constant receiving of His Spirit, a life of unreserved surrender to His service. The channel of communication must be open continually between man and his God. As the vine branch constantly draws the sap from the living vine, so are we to cling to Jesus, and receive from Him by faith the strength and perfection of His own character."[297]

In choosing Christ, and putting our faith in Him, we are connected with the Vine, and His life becomes ours.

5. Search my heart

I search my heart to understand the motivation behind what I do, so that the deception of my heart dies in the light of God's love, and I can intelligently surrender the revealed defects of my heart to

---

[297] White, E. G. (1898) *The Desire of Ages*. (p 675-6). Review and Herald Publishing Association.

Christ that He may be able to overcome those defects and replace them with victory in and through His power.

6. Choose to Think Only Positively About Them

I think only good thoughts about others.

"The soul can be in a state of peace only by relying upon God, and by partaking of the divine nature through faith in the Son of God. The Spirit of God produces a new life in the soul, bringing the thoughts and desires into obedience to the will of Christ, and the inward man is renewed in the image of Him who works in us to subdue all things unto himself. As God works upon the heart by his Holy Spirit, man must co-operate with him. The thoughts must be bound about, restricted, withdrawn from branching out and contemplating things that will only weaken and defile the soul. The thoughts must be pure, the meditations of the heart must be clean, if the words of the mouth are to be words acceptable to Heaven, and helpful to your associates...In the sermon on the mount, Christ presented before his disciples the far-reaching principles of the law of God. He taught his hearers that the law was transgressed by the thoughts before the evil desire was carried out in actual commission. We are under obligation to control our thoughts, and to bring them into subjection to the law of God. The noble powers of the mind have been given to us by the Lord, that we may employ them in contemplating heavenly things."[298]

By God's grace I can think well of even those who hurt me.

7. Love Others

I have the privilege of giving to others the love that I took from God.

"When self is merged in Christ, love springs forth spontaneously. The completeness of Christian character is attained

---

[298] White, E. G. The Renewing of the Mind. *The Review and Herald.* June 12, 1888, paragraph 3.

when the impulse to help and bless others springs constantly from within—when the sunshine of heaven fills the heart and is revealed in the countenance."[299]

Love for God automatically springs forth in love to others.

8. Remember, It's Not Mine

I need to remind myself, "It's not mine!" I don't possess it. I can't produce it. I am not my own. I am just the delivery guy. It is all God's.

9. Use Natural Remedies, Change My Lifestyle

I use natural remedies, and I change my lifestyle to fit that which God delights in, because I love Him.

10. Get (Back) Up

I get up and get back up. I make the effort, and He provides the power.

If I would have given this 10-part prescription to you at the beginning of this series, would you have accepted it, or thrown it away? Would you have believed me that these points are vitally important to your physical health? Or, would you have gone in search for a second opinion? I pray that you now see that these points are vitally important to your health and healing—of body, mind, and soul.

A number of years ago, I fell in love with the following quote. "When the gospel is received in its purity and power, it is a cure for the maladies that originated in sin."[301] Which maladies originated in sin? Diabetes? Heart disease? Cancer? Obesity? Arthritis? Auto-immune diseases? All maladies originated in sin. And what is a cure

[299] White, E. G. (1900) *Christ's Object Lessons.* (p 384). Review and Herald Publishing Association.
[301] White, E. G. (1905) *The Ministry of Healing.* (p. 115) Mountain View, CA: Pacific Press Publishing Association.

for the maladies that originated in sin? The gospel received in its purity and power is that cure.

The Law of Life

So, what is the Law of Life? "...the principles of righteousness embodied in the Decalogue are as immutable as the eternal throne. Not one command has been annulled, not a jot or tittle has been changed. Those principles that were made known to man in Paradise as the great **law of life** will exist unchanged in Paradise restored. When Eden shall bloom on earth again, God's law of love will be obeyed by all beneath the sun."[303] The Law of God is the law of life.

"God's wonderful purpose of grace, the mystery of redeeming love, is the theme into which "angels desire to look," and it will be their study throughout endless ages. Both the redeemed and the unfallen beings will find in the cross of Christ their science and their song. It will be seen that the glory shining in the face of Jesus is the glory of self-sacrificing love. In the light from Calvary it will be seen that the law of self-renouncing love is **the law of life** for earth and heaven; that the love which "seeketh not her own" has its source in the heart of God; and that in the meek and lowly One is manifested the character of Him who dwelleth in the light which no man can approach unto."[304] The Law of Life is self-renouncing love.

"Looking unto Jesus we see that it is the glory of our God to give. 'I do nothing of Myself,' said Christ...'I seek not Mine own glory,' but the glory of Him that sent Me. John 8:28; 6:57; 8:50; 7:18. In these words is set forth the great principle which is **the law of life** for the universe. All things Christ received from God, but **He took to give.** So in the heavenly courts, in His ministry for all created beings: through the beloved Son, the Father's life flows out to all; through the

[303] White, E. G. (1896) *Thoughts from the Mount of Blessing.* (p 50). Mountain View, CA: Pacific Press Publishing Association.
[304] White, E. G. (1898) *The Desire of Ages.* (p 19). Review and Herald Publishing Association.

Son it returns, in praise and joyous service, a tide of love, to the great Source of all. And thus through Christ the circuit of beneficence is complete, representing the character of the great Giver, **the law of life**."[305]

"All things both in heaven and in earth declare that the great **law of life** is a law of service. The infinite Father ministers to the life of every living thing. Christ came to the earth 'as He that serveth.' The angels are 'ministering spirits, sent forth to minister for them who shall be heirs of salvation.' The same law of service is written upon all things in nature. The birds of the air, the beasts of the field, the trees of the forest, the leaves, the grass, and the flowers, the sun in the heavens and the stars of light—all have their ministry. Lake and ocean, river and water spring—**each takes to give**."[306] The Law of Life is the law of service, taking to give. And that Law of Life, applied to one's life, brings health and life and love.

[305] White, E. G. (1898) *The Desire of Ages*. (p 21). Review and Herald Publishing Association.
[306] White, E. G. (1903) *Education*. (p 103). Mountain View, CA: Pacific Press Publishing Association.

FINAL SUMMARY

We were created in the image of God, which means that we were created to think like God thinks. We were also created with a need for love, of which God is the only source. God is unselfish, so, to function as God created us, we unselfishly come to Him, taking of His love and giving it away to others, just as His 10-commandment law shows us. When we think as God thinks, unselfishly taking of His love in order to give it away to others, that provides the power and control that the cells of the body need in order to function properly. True health can only be expected if we are functioning according to how we were created.

When man sinned and broke that 10-commandment law, we became unimaginably deceived. We came to believe that we are god, that we are owners, that others "owe" us, but also that others are our source of love. In our deception, we became slaves to others even as we tried to control them. We accepted a false "love," which is actually selfishness, that gives in order to receive. The old heart with its up-side-down thinking and uncontrollable losses became our reality.

That old, sinful heart can never comply with God's law and can never think as God thinks. Also, in sin, we accept a substitute for love which is no love at all. Since our thinking is not aligned with God's thinking, and since we accept a substitute for love which is not love, this results in the wrong power and control of the cells of our body, and disease and dysfunction is the result.

God knew that we were helplessly lost in the deception of sin, so He sent Jesus to rescue us from our hopeless situation. Because of the infinite gift of God through Jesus, He gives us the chance to have a new heart—His heart—which is in harmony with His law and is restored to the original creation. As this new heart is restored in us, our thinking aligns with God's thinking, and we come to Him as our only source of all things, including love. This restoration contributes to 90% of our health and healing, although we are still subject to inheritance, environment, raw materials, and the enemy's attacks.

The new heart, which is a product of God's grace, not only promotes physical health. It also gives us peace in all situations and circumstances. It saves us from taking things personally. It gives us joy in believing the truth. It restores relationships that have been broken through the craziness of sin. I want that new heart! Don't you? God wants it for you too. Remember, He died so that you could have it.

Improving Health...
One Choice At A Time

UCHEE PINES INSTITUTE

Uchee Pines Institute is an educational and religious charitable organization designed to help those suffering from disease and the effects of faulty lifestyle, as well as to train medical missionary lay workers to perpetuate the methods of health evangelism and simple remedies for disease.

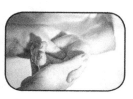

◆ Lifestyle Center
We offer a 17-day residential experience in health education and lifestyle change. If you're chronically sick, in pain, stressed, battling cancer, dealing with diabetes, concerned about high blood pressure, or just eager to learn about health, then you need to come. Renew your health – for good!

◆ Health Education
Uchee Pines is known worldwide for its dynamic and informative health and wellness seminars. Some we provide are:
Simple Remedies and Preventive Medicine – Combine practical, lifestyle education, with spiritual renewal and hands-on training in only 4 days!
Health Emphasis Weekend (HEW) – Tailored for your local church/area, HEWs are effective in both educating the members and providing a means of evangelism for your community.
Continuing Education Credits – The only Christian lifestyle and natural remedies-focused seminar that offers CME's/CEU's for healthcare professionals.

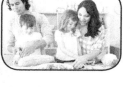

◆ Missionary Training & Health Evangelism
This program seeks to produce self-sacrificing missionaries with the ability to support themselves and their mission projects and serve the Lord and their fellow man through medical missionary work. Come to our campus and become a **Lifestyle Educator** and **Lifestyle Counselor**.

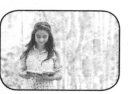

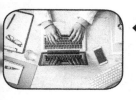

◆ Lifestyle Counselling and Coaching
We offer Outpatient and Phone Consultations for those who cannot come to the facility. Our website Counseling Sheets are one of the largest online sources of natural health information available. Through books, DVDs, and the Uchee Pines YouTube channel, we are able to come right to the home of people across the world, bringing spiritual and physical restoration.

If you are interested in coming to Uchee Pines, or hosting our team of health evangelists in your area, please contact us:

334-855-4764 | ucheepines.org

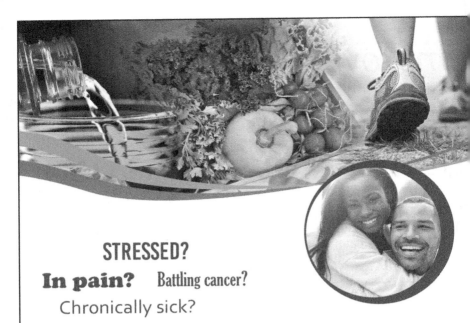

STRESSED?

In pain? Battling cancer?

Chronically sick?

DEALING WITH DIABETES? Struggling with arthritis?

TIME TO GET YOUR LIFESTYLE BACK ON TRACK?
Concerned about high blood pressure?

HAVING CHOLESTEROL ISSUES? **NEED A BREAK?**
Looking to lose weight?

IF YOU ANSWERED YES TO ANY OF THESE QUESTIONS
THEN YOU NEED TO COME TO UCHEE PINES! DON'T WAIT.
IMPROVE YOUR HEALTH ONE CHOICE AT A TIME.

CALL TODAY

877-UCHEEPINES

334-855-4764 • UCHEEPINES.ORG

Made in the USA
Monee, IL
11 May 2024

58055333R00157